W0050221

Workshop on
URSODEOXYCHOLIC ACID

Workshop on
URSODEOXYCHOLIC ACID

Workshop held in Cortina d'Ampezzo, March 1978

Editors

R. H. Dowling   A. F. Hofmann

Gastroenterology Unit,   Department of Medicine,
Guy's Hospital Medical School, University of California at
London, England   San Diego, California, USA

L. Barbara

Department of Gastroenterology,
Policlinico S. Orsola and School
of Medicine, University of Bologna, Italy

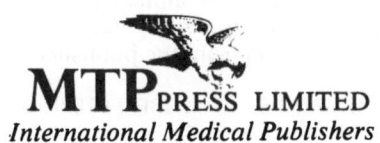

MTPPRESS LIMITED
International Medical Publishers

Published by
MTP Press Limited
Falcon House
Lancaster, England

Copyright © 1978 MTP Press Limited
Softcover reprint of the hardcover 1st edition 1978

All rights reserved. No part of this publication
may be reproduced, stored in a retrieval
system, or transmitted in any form or by any
means, electronic, mechanical, photocopying,
recording or otherwise, without prior
permission from the publishers.

ISBN 978-94-015-7284-2   ISBN 978-94-015-7282-8 (eBook)
DOI 10.1007/978-94-015-7282-8

foreword

Until ten years ago, the only treatment for gallstones was surgery. Now there is an effective alternative and, in suitable patients, gallstones can be dissolved with bile acid therapy. To date, most gallstone patients treated medically have been given chenodeoxycholic acid, but in 1974 another naturally occurring bile acid, ursodeoxycholic acid (which is structurally closely related to chenodeoxycholic acid), was introduced from Japan as a gallstone dissolving agent. Since then, its use has spread to the West and already many aspects of the physiology, biochemistry, pharmacology, toxicity and efficacy of 'urso' have been studied. As is often the case when a new therapeutic agent challenges the old, the question arose — will 'urso' replace 'cheno' as the medical treatment of choice for dissolving gallstones? To answer this and other related questions, the first ever workshop on ursodeoxycholic acid was held in Cortina, Italy during March 1978. Experts from both East and West met to discuss their latest results with ursodeoxycholic acid and to compare and contrast 'urso' and 'cheno'. The proceedings of this conference were recorded and appear here in edited form.

This workshop formed part of the IVth International Bile Acid Meeting organised by the University of Bologna and was sponsored by the Giuliani Company, Italy. The organisers wish to thank the Misses Margaret Henderson and Vicky Huebner for valuable secretarial assistance.

Hermon Dowling
Alan Hofmann
Luigi Barbara   *October 1978*

Foreword

Participants

BARBARA, Professor Luigi
Cattedra di Gastroenterologia, Policlinico S. Orsola, Via Massarenti 9, 40138 Bologna, Italy.

BAZZOLI, Dr Franco
Cattedra di Gastroenterologia, Policlinico S. Orsola, Via Massarenti 9, 40138 Bologna, Italy.

BONVICINI, Dr Fiorenza
Patologia Medica 3⁰, Policlinico S. Orsola, Via Massarenti 9, 40138 Bologna, Italy.

CACIAGLI, Professor Francesco
Cattedra di Farmacologia, Madonna delle Piane, Chieti, Italy.

CHADWICK, Dr Vinton
Department of Medicine, Royal Postgraduate Medical School, Hammersmith Hospital, London W12, England.

DOWLING, Professor R. Hermon
Gastroenterology Unit, Department of Medicine, Guy's Hospital Medical School, London, SE1 9RT, England.

FROMM, Dr Hans
University of Pittsburgh, Montefiore Hospital, Pittsburgh, Pennsylvania 15213, USA.

GASBARRINI, Professor Giovanni
Direttore Patologia Medica 3⁰, Policlinico S. Orsola, Via Massarenti 9, 40138 Bologna, Italy.

GRUNDY, Dr Scott
Department of Medicine, Veterans Administration Hospital, La Jolla, California 92037, USA.

HOFMANN, Professor Alan F.
Department of Medicine, University of California at San Diego, University Hospital Medical Center, 225 Dickinson Street, San Diego, California 92103, USA.

KRITCHEVSKY, Dr David
Associate Director, Wistar Institute of Anatomy and Biology, Philadelphia, Pennsylvania 19104, USA.

MATON, Dr Paul
Gastroenterology Unit, Guy's Hospital, London SE1 9RT, England.

MAZZELLA, Dr Giuseppe
Cattedra di Gastroenterologia, Policlinico S. Orsola, Via Massarenti 9, 40138 Bologna, Italy.

MIETTINEN, Dr Tatu
Third Department of Medicine, University of Helsinki, Helsinki 29, Finland.

OSUGA, Professor Toshiaki
Institute of Clinical Medicine, University of Tsukuba, Niihari-Gun, Ibaraki-Ken 300-31, Tokyo, Japan.

PODDA, Dr Mauro
Istituto di Clinica Medica 3°, Via Pace 15, Milano, Italy.

RODA, Dr Aldo
Cattedra di Chimica Gen. ed Inorg., Facoltà di Farmacia, Università di Bologna, Italy.

RODA, Dr Enrico
Cattedra di Gastroenterologia, Policlinico S. Orsola, Via Massarenti 9, 40138 Bologna, Italy.

SALEN, Professor Gerald
College of Medicine and Dentistry, New Jersey Medical School, 100 Bergen Street, Newark, New Jersey 07103, USA.

SALVIOLI, Dr Gianfranco
Istituto di Clinica Medica, Via del Pozzo 3, Modena, Italy.

SAMA, Dr Claudia
Cattedra di Gastroenterologia, Policlinico S. Orsola, Via Massarenti 9, 40138 Bologna, Italy.

STIEHL, Professor Adolf
Klinikum der Universität, Abteilung 1.1.4 - Innere Medizin IV, Berghemer Strasse 58, Heidelberg, West Germany.

THISTLE, Dr Johnson L.
Division of Gastroenterology, Mayo Clinic and Mayo Foundation, Rochester, Minnesota 55901, USA.

Workshop on Ursodeoxycholic Acid

Dowling: On behalf of my Co-chairmen, Professor Alan Hofmann from San Diego, California, and Professor Luigi Barbara from Bologna, I should like to welcome you to the first workshop on the subject of ursodeoxycholic acid (UDCA). We hope that the decision to publish the proceedings of this workshop will not in any way inhibit a free and open discussion or the presentation of results of work which is still in progress.

Last year in Milan at a meeting organized by Professor Dioguardi, we listed some of the substances which are known to reduce the saturation of bile with cholesterol and/or to dissolve gallstones (Figure 1). No less than five of these are bile acids which have been used either alone or in combination with other substances. Today we are concerned with the fourth item on the list, UDCA. We all owe a debt of gratitude to our colleagues from Japan where the substance has been used as a choleretic for many years. In particular I think we should acknowledge the valuable contribution of Isao Makino and his colleagues (1975) who first showed that UDCA, like chenodeoxycholic acid (CDCA), dissolves gallstones.

At the Milan meeting we also discussed some of the theoretical advantages and disadvantages of using UDCA (as opposed to CDCA) for gallstone dissolution (Figures 2 and 3). From the results of the Japanese studies, it seemed that UDCA was as effective as CDCA, but, in addition, it seemed to dissolve gallstones at a lower dose. In a paper published in *The Lancet,* Nagakawa *et al.* (1977) found

BILE ACIDS	OTHERS
1. **CHENODEOXYCHOLIC ACID** (Thistle & Schoenfield, 1971)	6. **SOYA BEAN LECITHIN** (Tompkins et al, 1970)
2. **CDCA + PHENOBARB** (Coyne et al, 1975)	7. **β-GLYCEROPHOSPHATE** (Linscheer & Raheja,1974)
3. **CDCA + β-SITOSTEROL** (Gerolami & Sarles, 1975)	8. **PHENOBARB** (Redinger & Small, 1973)
– – – – – – – – – – – – – 4. **URSODEOXYCHOLIC ACID** (Makino et al, 1975)	9. **"ZANCHOL"** (FLORANTYRONE) (Kirkpatrick et al, 1974)
5. **CHOLIC ACID + LECITHIN** (Toouli et al, 1975)	10. **BRAN** (Pomare & Heaton, 1973)

Figure 1 Substances claimed to reduce the saturation of bile in cholesterol and/or to dissolve cholesterol-rich gallstones

1) Effective in lower doses than CDCA

   - with 150mg ($2.9mg.kgBW^{-1}day^{-1}$) dissoln. in 6/16 at 6 months

    - Nakagawa, Makino et al (1977)

2) No hypertransaminaseaemia

3) Does not affect colonic mucosal ultrastructure
    - Chadwick et al (1976)

  Does not provoke colonic H_2O secretion

    - Debongnie and Phillips (1977)

∴ May not cause diarrhoea

4) Lowers serum triglycerides by 21%
    - Nakagawa et al (1977)

Figure 2 Apparent advantages of using UDCA (rather than CDCA) for the treatment of patients with presumed cholesterol gallstones (mid-1977)

that at doses as low as 2.9 mg/kg, UDCA effectively dissolved gallstones and did not provoke any increase in serum transaminase levels. Furthermore, UDCA does not affect colonic mucosal ultrastructure - at least in rabbits (Chadwick *et al.*, 1976a) - nor does it provoke colonic water secretion (Debongnie and Phillips, 1977). For these reasons, it was thought that UDCA might not cause diarrhea, and this has certainly been borne out by the initial clinical results. In several studies, there was also the suggestion that UDCA lowers fasting serum triglycerides to a greater extent and more consistently than CDCA.

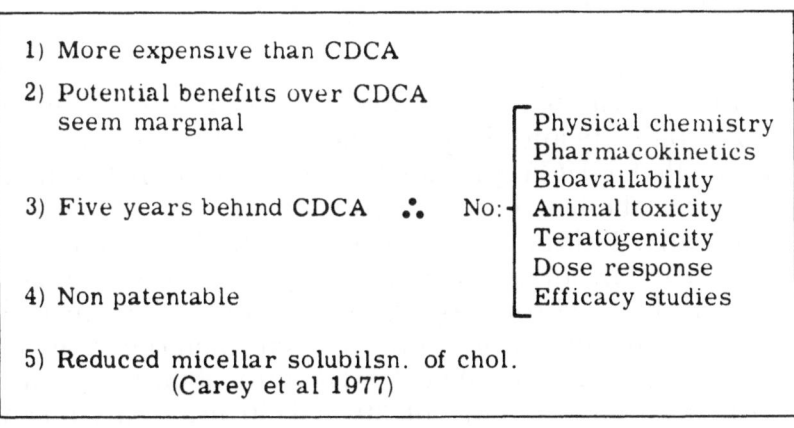

Figure 3 Apparent disadvantages of using UDCA (rather than CDCA) for the treatment of patients with presumed cholesterol gallstones (mid-1977)

But from a commercial point of view there were also disadvantages. Since UDCA is synthesized from CDCA, it is more expensive to manufacture, and at the time of the Milan meeting at least, it seemed that the potential benefits of UDCA over CDCA were marginal. Whether or not that is still the case is the *raison d'etre* of today's meeting.

UDCA is about 5 years behind CDCA in its development. For that reason, the basic studies of physical chemistry, pharmacokinetics, bioavailability, etc., have not yet been carried out by pharmaceutical companies.

Such studies are expensive, and since UDCA, like CDCA, is another naturally-occurring bile acid, it is a non-patentable compound. However, such considerations should not inhibit us from pursuing our clinical investigations with UDCA.

Finally, there was the suggestion made by Martin Carey (1977) that UDCA is not such a good detergent as other major bile acids and that the micellar solubilization of cholesterol is less in UDCA-rich bile than in mixed micellar solutions containing other bile acids.

With that brief introduction, let us start by considering the bioavailability, pharmacology, and pharmaco-kinetics of UDCA.

Sama: I wish to present our preliminary data on the bioavailability and the pharmacology of UDCA. We used unlabelled UDCA provided by the Giuliani Company and ^{3}H-labelled UDCA provided by the Amersham Company. This labeled UDCA was found to be impure by thin-layer chromatography, so we purified the ^{3}H-UDCA by thin-layer chromatography, checking the purity by zonal scanning. The pure labeled material was co-crystallized with unlabeled UDCA to obtain a product with a specific activity of 30 μCi/30 mg. This labeled UDCA was packed in gelatin capsules together with unlabeled UDCA. Table 1 shows data describing the

Table 1   Area under the curve (AUC_0), based on serum radioactivity, after oral administration of varying doses of UDCA together with ^{3}H-UDCA (30 μCi) in six normal subjects

UDCA (mg)	^{3}H-UDCA (μCi)	AUC_0 (% dose $\times 10^{-2} \times 4$ h)
300	30	8.5
300	30	14.1
150	30	13.5
150	30	18.3
75	30	18.2
75	30	7.9

appearance of radioactivity in peripheral blood, expressed as area under the curve, after oral administration of 30 μCi of ³H-UDCA with varying amounts of unlabeled UCDA (75, 150 and 300 mg). Six subjects were each studied on three occasions, with a different dose given each time. The fraction of the absorbed dose appearing in peripheral blood was constant for each group of subjects, indicating that intestinal absorption and hepatic clearance were constant and apparently unrelated to dose.

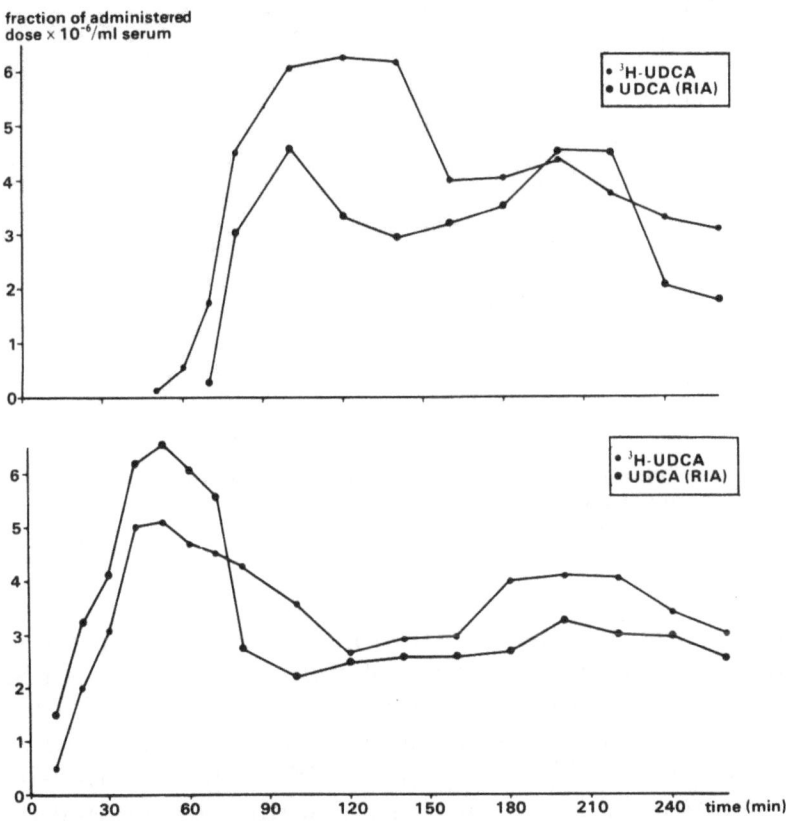

Figure 4 Appearance of ³H-ursodeoxycholic acid (³H-UDCA) and un-labeled UDCA in peripheral blood in two individual subjects (upper and lower panel) after ingestion of a gelatin capsule containing 300 mg UDCA and 30 mg of ³H-UDCA (30 μCi)

Our results were similar, whether calculated from chemical concentration or radioactivity (Figure 4). To measure the chemical concentration of UDCA in serum, we used a radioimmunoassay developed by Dr Aldo Roda in our laboratory (Roda *et al.*, in preparation). In Figure 5, we show the appearance of radioactivity in peripheral

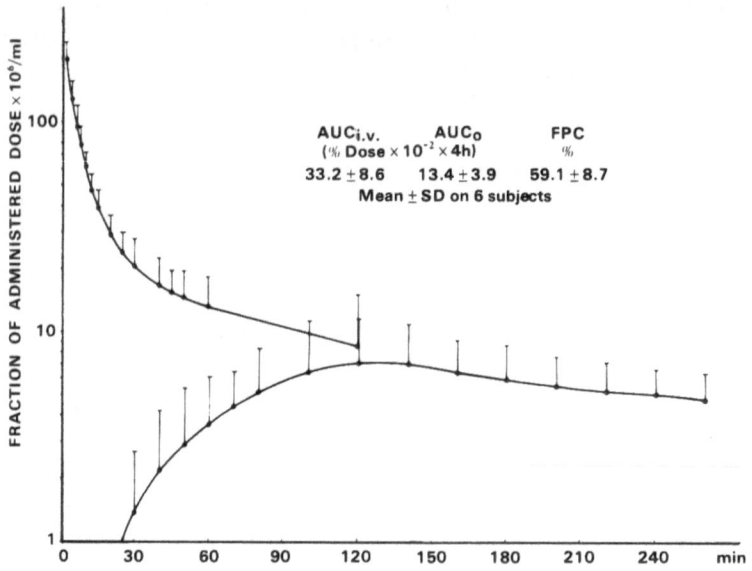

Figure 5 Plasma disappearance of radioactivity after intravenous administration of ³H-UDCA and plasma appearance of radioactivity after oral administration of ³H-UDCA. The data are the mean (±SD) for studies in six subjects. Studies were carried out 2 weeks apart

blood after oral administration of ³H-UDCA, as well as the plasma disappearance of radioactivity (Mean ± SD) after intravenous injection of ³H-UDCA. We have measured first-pass clearance by the conventional equation: $(1 - AUC_o/AUC_{i.v.}) \times 100$. The mean first-pass clearance (59.1 ± 8.7) was quite similar to the first-pass clearance of CDCA measured by Drs van Berge Henegouwen and Hofmann (1977b). Thus, we conclude that UDCA is well absorbed. Indeed, since the proportion of UDCA appearing in peripheral blood is constant and

14

unrelated to dose, it appears that UDCA is completely absorbed.

Hofmann: These are very nice studies, and I fully agree with Dr Sama's conclusions. Dr van Berge Henegouwen's bioavailability studies were difficult to design properly. It is not a simple problem to assess the bioavailability of substances such as CDCA and UDCA which have a large first-pass clearance. What Dr van Berge Henegouwen did was to infuse different amounts of the sodium salt into the intestine to get a calibration curve which related the amount absorbed to the AUC of the serum level curve. Dr Sama is also planning to use this approach.

Her data, nonetheless, are certainly consistent with the view that UDCA is fully bioavailable.

Has anyone carried out any dissolution studies to compare UDCA with CDCA?

(Negative response)

Do we have any estimate of the first-pass clearance of UDCA?

Sama: Our data give a figure of 60%.

Hofmann: Well certainly Dr Sama's studies suggest that bioavailability of UDCA will not be a problem. Thus, since both CDCA and UDCA are fully bioavailable, the problems of bacterial biotransformation apply only after either compound has left the enterohepatic circulation.

Dowling: Dr Sama, if I may clarify one point, did you establish 'reference' serum concentration time curves by infusing solutions of bile acids directly into the intestine and proving that they had been completely absorbed?

Sama: No.

Dowling: I suspect that this would be necessary to validate your results. Such validation also depends on the reliability of the duodenal infusion technique as a means of obtaining a 100% bioavailable reference curve comparable to that obtained by intravenous injection of other drugs. Using the duodenal infusion technique, Dr Ponz de Leon in our Unit found somewhat different results from the Mayo Clinic data for CDCA bioavailability (Ponz de Leon *et al.*, 1977).

In the method used in these studies, one infuses a solution containing ^{3}H-labeled bile acid and ^{14}C-labeled polyethylene glycol (PEG) into the duodenum and then analyzes the ^{3}H/^{14}C ratio in intestinal contents aspirated from sites distal to the infusion port. In the Mayo studies, I believe that this was 50 cm downstream, whereas Dr Ponz de Leon sampled from two sites - at 60 and 120 cm downstream from the infusion port. Because we gave a bolus injection of bile acid plus PEG (as opposed to the steady-state situation with a constant infusion technique), we could not measure recovery quantitatively. The validity of the duodenal bolus infusion technique as a means for providing a reference standard against which the bioavailability of orally ingested capsules and tablets can be compared, relies entirely on 100% absorption of the duodenally infused bile acids. One has to demonstrate, therefore, that there is never any bile acid and that the ^{14}C/^{3}H ratio is always infinity at the distal sampling site to prove complete absorption. In our experience, this was not the case, even at 120 cm downstream from the infusion port.

There are ways to overcome this problem, and Dr Ponz de Leon, working in Dr Carulli's department, has been extending the work carried out with us in London by doing further studies here in Italy. Would Dr Carulli care to comment?

Carulli: I am not completely familiar with the data, but in Modena Dr Ponz de Leon has now completed his studies of CDCA bioavailability which he carried out in London when he was working at Guy's, with Professor Dowling. Briefly, his studies showed that when given in gelatin-coated capsules, CDCA was solubilized into the enteric secretions and its solubility seemed to be strictly dependent on the luminal pH and, to a lesser extent, on the concentration of endogenous bile acids. In addition, when three different doses of CDCA were given to the same volunteers both as capsules and as intraduodenal aqueous solutions, bioavailability was complete (as may be deduced from the comparison of the areas under the concentration-time curves) up to 500 mg doses, but fell to approximately 70%, in most of the subjects studied, with the higher dose (750 mg). As far as intestinal absorption of the infused CDCA is concerned, his studies seem to indicate that, when given as a bolus, most of the infused CDCA is rapidly absorbed over 120 cm of intestine (95-98% of the dose, when an occluding balloon and a non-absorbable marker are used).

Hofmann: Ten years ago, in my first work at the Mayo Clinic, Ian Hislop and I carried out steady-state perfusions with micellar solutions and found the absorption of CDCA in a 50 cm test segment to be about 90% (Hislop *et al.*, 1967). I therefore continue to believe that any sampling will show rapid passive absorption of CDCA.

If one takes a capsule greater than 400 mg, then I am perfectly prepared to say that there can be a problem of kinetics of dissolution in relation to intestinal transit. Our data can only be applied to a single 400 mg dose. For a higher dose, we do not have data. Therefore, it is clear that single, higher doses are well absorbed, but I cannot say that they are 100%.

Dowling: The CDCA doses which we used were 250, 500 and 750 mg. Our lowest dose is therefore below your 400 mg dose, and, even then, we could not prove 100% intestinal absorption of the duodenally infused material. In our opinion, it is not adequate to say that 90% or more was absorbed: if 100% absorption has not been proven, one cannot use the resultant systemic serum CDCA concentration time curves as reference standards.

But we should not prolong this discussion; we are supposed to be talking about UDCA and not about CDCA.

Hofmann: In my opinion, the isotope dilution technique of Lindstedt (1957), as reported by us, has a dangerous degree of uncertainty in patients ingesting large doses of bile acids. I do not think now that one can accurately calculate absorption of ingested bile acids using this technique, as we reported in the original paper by Danzinger *et al.* (1972). In some patients ingesting bile acids, we recently obtained input figures which far exceed the daily dosage of ingested bile acids (Tangedahl *et al.*, 1978 (in press)). I am not sure why this is. I suppose one possibility is a large, slowly equilibrating pool of bile acids in the colon.

Stiehl: Why does Professor Hofmann feel that the Lindstedt technique is inaccurate?

Hofmann: I do not want to discuss the Lindstedt technique in general. I only want to say in a new set of studies in which bile acid kinetics were measured in patients receiving oral cholic and CDCA, our calculated input figures, using the Lindstedt technique, did not agree with the oral dose. And these studies were done very carefully. We got figures that were much too high. I do not know why, but that is what we got.

Salen: One problem that may explain this discrepancy concerns the effect of intestinal bacteria on the ingested bile acid. In other words, feeding bile acids into the body and exposing them to the bacterial flora results in considerable degradation of the bile acid and may affect the bile acid turnover curves, especially if equilibrium was not attained.

Therefore, when we fed a gram per day of bile acid, we had no way of knowing the proportion of that gram of bile acid that was destroyed or that entered the pool. However, despite this reservation, I think the data are interesting - but must be interpreted cautiously.

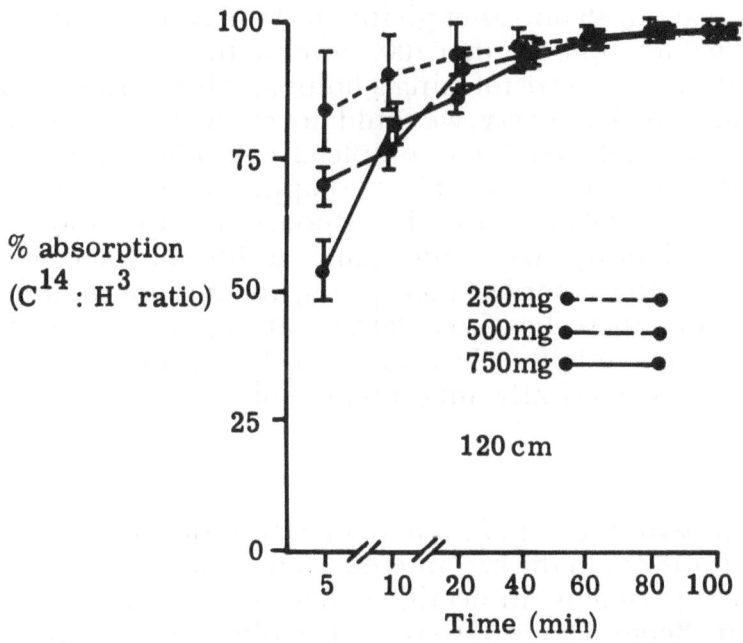

Figure 6 Intestinal 'absorption' of three different doses of ^{3}H-labeled CDCA from duodenal bolus infusions of aqueous solutions containing the sodium salt of the bile acid and ^{14}C-PEG (as a non-absorbable marker). Results are plotted as 'percentage absorption' of the infused dose, calculated from the ^{14}C/^{3}H ratios in intestinal contents aspirated 120 cm distal to the infusion port for the 250, 500 and 750 mg CDCA doses. (From Ponz de Leon *et al.* 1977, *Gut,* **18,** A976).

Hofmann: We are talking about the steady-state pharmacology of UDCA when we should be discussing its pharmacokinetics.

Dowling: We should not dwell on this, but Figure 6 illustrates some results from Dr Ponz de Leon's studies (1977) showing the ratio of ^{14}C-labeled PEG to ^{3}H-labeled bile acid, 120 cm distal to the infusion site in the duodenum, when control subjects were given 250, 500 and 750 mg of ^{3}H-labeled CDCA. If all the CDCA had been absorbed, then no ^{3}H would have appeared at the distal sampling site, the ^{14}C/^{3}H ratio would have been infinity, indicating 100% bile acid absorption. However, it was not until about 40 min after giving the bolus infusion that we started to approach that 100% level in the distal aspirates. And since we were infusing a bolus and had no idea about quantitative recovery, we could not say with certainty that the material had been completely absorbed. The same objection would probably also apply if we had infused labeled UDCA into the duodenum to study its bioavailability with the same technique. We must demonstrate complete absorption, and it is not enough to say that there has been 90-95% absorption, since that represents only the absorption on the aspirated material which, theoretically, might represent no more than 5% of the infused load.

Hofmann: We found more than 99% absorption. I believe that it is not in the best interests of this meeting to discuss our experiments in detail, as they are already published (van Berge Henegouwen and Hofmann, 1977b). We should meet privately to work out our disagreements.

Salen: We fed unlabeled UDCA to patients at a dose of 1 g daily. After 2 weeks of UDCA feeding, they were given an intravenous pulse-label of 24-^{14}C-UDCA. The specific activity of biliary UDCA obtained for the 5 days after pulse-labeling. showed a linear decay suggesting a single pool of UDCA in the enterohepatic circulation.

I should like to emphasize that UDCA was converted also in part to CDCA. We found that the specific activity of biliary CDCA rose during the experiment, so that there is some interconversion between UDCA and CDCA.

It is also possible to calculate UDCA pool size and production rates from mathematical analyses of the decay curves which, in the case of UDCA, should give a figure for the absorption of UDCA. When we calculated this, we found that approximately 90% of the daily dose of UDCA entered the exchangeable pool and that the pool turned over very rapidly (Fedorowski *et al.*, 1977).

Hofmann: When bioavailability studies are done, the UDCA is absorbed in unconjugated form. We should see the spillover of unconjugated UDCA in peripheral blood. There is no immediate conversion to CDCA.

I think - and perhaps Dr Sama has some data - that one will not find any label in CDCA until it has had time to pass into the distal intestine and be exposed to bacteria, which can oxidize it to 3-hydroxy-7-keto-lithocholic acid. When this is absorbed and reaches the liver, it will be reduced largely to CDCA, as shown in recent studies from Dr Fromm's laboratory (Fromm *et al.*, 1977; Fromm *et al.*, 1978).

I think that the initial radioactivity in blood will all be unconjugated UDCA.

Sama: Yes, in our studies serum radioactivity was present solely as unconjugated UDCA.

Salen: I agree that time is important. However, it is difficult to interpret acute experiments when equilibrium conditions have not been attained. When equilibrium has

21

not been reached, the bile acid pool may not be saturated with labeled bile acid, and consequently, the spillover into the peripheral circulation will not reflect the bile acid pool.

Dowling: That is a valid point, and it may well be that bioavailability, as measured by the techniques already discussed, might be quite different in patients who are on long-term treatment from those who are just starting therapy. So far, the experiments have been done mainly in control subjects given single CDCA doses.

Hofmann: I am sorry, but I do not agree, at least for CDCA. What was done with CDCA was to study gallstone patients on long term therapy with CDCA. We then gave them one dose of CDCA intravenously (^{14}C) and a second dose orally (^{3}H) and looked at the ratio of specific activity in bile. The ratio should have become identical if there was complete absorption of the oral dose, and indeed it became so. If my recollection is correct, we studied three patients who had been on CDCA for some time because we thought that this question should be answered (van Berge Henegouwen and Hofmann, 1977b).

Fromm: What would be an acceptable criterion for total absorption in a study in which intestinal contents from the distal end of a perfused intestinal segment are analyzed? Can total absorption be assumed only if no radioactivity of the infused label is recovered?

Dowling: Yes. I think it would depend on that. Since a bolus duodenal infusion was given, and since one has no idea about quantitative recovery, even if only 5% of the labeled bile acid that was infused is recovered at the distal sampling site, this could represent 5% of *all* the bile acid that was infused, or it could represent 5% of only 1% of the duodenally infused bile acid bolus. There is no way of being sure about this when one examines only the distal sampling site. If one had chosen a segmental perfusion technique, then having established a steady state, one could quantitate absorption and hopefully prove that it was 100%. But with this technique, significant amounts of the substrate are removed from the gut lumen (for analysis) which would otherwise have been available for absorption which thereby influences the serum concentration-time reference curve in the peripheral blood.

There are ways to overcome this problem which are being explored in our unit at present.

Fromm: Do you feel that the constant perfusion technique is the only acceptable method? I am sorry, but I shall have to ask you to be more specific, since you labour this point.

Dowling: Yes. When Dr John Fordtran visited us, he made a valuable suggestion. He suggested that we should use a constant duodenal infusion technique of an isotonic solution of sodium chloride containing mannitol (to inhibit water absorption) and PEG until steady-state conditions are reached. Then one should 'ride' the bile acid in as a bolus infusion on the back of the saline infusion in order to obtain, by deconvolutional analysis, a curve which would then demonstrate, hopefully, complete absorption. But one needs to do this to obtain quantitative measures of recovery - not just spot samples, which is what we have been doing so far.

Fromm: We have indeed obtained a continuous collection and not just a spot sample at the distal site of the infused segment. I have discussed this problem of the interpretation of the results of a bolus infusion with Dr S. Adibi in our unit who applies similarly strict criteria as Dr Fordtran. He pointed out that even when there is no recovery of radioactivity at the distal end of the segment, he would not accept this as a reliable criterion for complete absorption. Therefore, this particular question remains a problem.

Dowling: Anyone who intends to do serious bioavailability studies with UDCA will have the same problems, and these technical problems must be sorted out before the methods can really be validated. Perhaps we also need more information about bioavailability in patients who are on long-term bile acid treatment as well as in control subjects - and perhaps not just with tracer doses of isotope which, I think, was the basis of Dr Thistle and Dr Hofmann's studies - or did you give the 400 mg of CDCA intravenously?

Hofmann: No. But we have certainly done it with cholic acid, and there is no difference between the clearance of intravenously injected tracer and 400 mg (Calcraft *et al.*, 1975). One probably cannot give 400 mg of CDCA intravenously. It would induce considerable hemolysis.

Dowling: Nor can we do the same thing with UDCA, so we cannot resolve that particular problem.

Hofmann: Occasionally in science we must use strong inference. There is really no reason to believe that the first-pass clearance of 400 mg will be different from tracer. All the animal work agrees in finding that the V_{max} for hepatic transport for bile acids is very high (Erlinger *et al.*, 1977; Reichen *et al.*, 1977).

24

Dowling: That might well be right, but we cannot prove it.

Even though we have been quibbling about minor details, it seems probable that UDCA, like CDCA, will be highly bioavailable.

Hofmann: Could we ask whether anyone has information on the pH solubility curve of UDCA compared to CDCA? I have not done that experiment, and I should like to know the answer. The solubility of CDCA goes up strikingly above pH 6.4-6.6, and it becomes very soluble (van Berge Henegouwen *et al.*, 1977a). So I wonder if anyone has determined the pH solubility curve of CDCA.

(No response)

Dowling: So nobody has *in vitro* studies on this, and nobody has put a tube down the intestine to sample contents and relate the solubility of UDCA in aspirated material to ambient intestinal pH at different sites? No? Then this is an experiment for all of us to do.

The next topic was raised by Martin Carey's interesting observations (1977) which implied that UDCA was a rather poor detergent and that it solubilized both lipid and cholesterol less well than other bile acids. Dr Helmut Greim also noted that UDCA had less effect than CDCA on Cytochrome P450 enzymes.

As far as I know, Dr Chadwick is the only person here to have worked on this specific problem by studying lipid solubility *in vivo* in patients taking UDCA.

Chadwick: In experiments carried out in collaboration with Dr van Berge Henegouwen in Holland, UDCA was fed to four normal volunteers at a dose of 1 g, in divided doses daily. We looked at the bile acid and fatty acid concentrations in the micellar phase after a liquid test meal, according to established techniques. We found that the average bile acid concentration for the 2-hour period following the liquid meal was 6.1 mmol/l during the control period and 6.6 mmol/l during UDCA therapy. (This difference was not significant.) The peak bile acid concentrations were also comparable, as were the fatty acid concentrations. The proportion of UDCA in the micellar bile acids was of the order of 62%, and that was all conjugated.

What can we say? It appears that there are good concentrations of bile acids in the micellar phase and a good concentration of lipids in normal subjects. Whether that means that UDCA is an adequate micelle former, compared to CDCA, I should not like to say until more *in vitro* studies have been done.

Hofmann: There are two factors. What one does in an experiment like this is to measure the distribution ratio between the oil phase and the micellar phase? Even though UDCA might be a poor solubilizer of monoglyceride and fatty acid, being a dihydroxy acid, it would have a lower critical micellization concentration than cholate, and the two might balance each other out.

I am pleased to see these results. They are perhaps predictable, but it is very good to have them shown experimentally.

Fromm: In cooperation with Dr Cussler and Dr Evans from the Department of Chemical Engineering at the Carnegie Mellon University of Pittsburgh, we have compared the dissolution rate of cholesterol in solution of UDCA or CDCA, using the spinning disc technique (Shaeiwitz *et al.*, 1977). This technique permits the study of the rate of dissolution of cholesterol at different speeds of the spinning disc. We found that UDCA effects only a slightly smaller dissolution rate than CDCA. Dissolution rate is not to be confused with solubility. They are different measurements.

Dowling: Dissolution of the bile acids themselves?

Fromm: No. Dissolution of a disc consisting of cholesterol.

Dowling: In other words, this is the dissolution of cholesterol in either UDCA or CDCA?

Fromm: The dissolution studies were carried out in bile acid-lecithin solutions. Lecithin was found to decrease the rate of cholesterol dissolution. I don't have the data with me, but they have been published in abstract form in *Clinical Research* (Shaeiwitz *et al.*, 1977).

Dowling: So in summary, UDCA solubilizes cholesterol a little less well -

Fromm: Not solubilizes. Dissolves. There is a difference.

Dowling: - a little less rapidly than CDCA in the presence of phospholipids.

Salen: Recently, Dr Igimi (1977) from Japan reported data for the solubility of cholesterol in pure UDCA-lecithin micelles and mixed UDCA-lecithin micellar solutions. When sodium tauro-ursodeoxycholate was used, the amount of cholesterol that was solubilized was considerably less than with sodium tauro-chenodeoxycholate. The conclusion from this paper was that UDCA should be a less effective gallstone dissolving agent.
However, one has to look at this experiment with a

different perspective. First is the fact that when UDCA is fed, about 50-60% of the bile acid is UDCA and there is a considerable amount of CDCA present in the bile. Further, looking at a pure system of UDCA does not accurately reflect the endogenous bile acid pool, even when UDCA is fed because considerable endogenous bile acid is present in the bile. Thus, the data on cholesterol solubilization with pure UDCA micelles may not reflect physiological conditions. However, another potential advantage of decreased cholesterol solubility in UDCA micelles is that less cholesterol may be absorbed from the intestines. This effect may increase the effectiveness of UDCA in reducing cholesterol saturation in the bile.

I would appreciate any comments on that point.

Hofmann: Let me restate the discussion. The independent observations of Igimi (1977) and Martin Carey (1977) indicate that the line in the triangle is lower in model systems when all the bile acids are replaced by UDCA. If that is true, then we can no longer calculate bile saturation using the equations of Paul Thomas (1973) or the technique suggested by Metzger *et al.* (1972).

Unfortunately, what no one has done since Holzbach *et al.* (1973) is to do what Johnston and Nakayama did (1957) - to define the actual cholesterol holding capacity of the bile samples in people taking UDCA to see whether or not it differs significantly from the Hegardt and Dam (1971) and Holzbach *et al.* (1973) lines.

The major difference between UDCA and CDCA, according to what I read, is that UDCA does not dissolve lecithin as well as CDCA, and accordingly, UDCA solutions, which are saturated with lecithin, dissolve less cholesterol than CDCA solutions saturated with lecithin.

So far, it looks as if this possible error in calculating the bile saturation of patients ingesting UDCA is not very important. Certainly patients with gallstones are responding to UDCA.

I think that we must take bile samples, determine the

biliary lipids, add cholesterol to achieve saturation, and determine the new cholesterol concentration. I think we should do it not only for people taking UDCA but even for people taking CDCA. The assumptions that we are making in calculating the change in saturation may not always be correct.

Dowling: I am sure that the differences here are fairly subtle. In November, 1977, Martin Carey was kind enough to send us information about the size of the correction factor in the saturation index for UDCA-rich bile. He suggested that the maximum error in saturation index was in the region of 8% in the Thomas-Hofmann polynomial (1973) - assuming that *all* bile acids which were present were UDCA conjugates, which, as we know from clinical experience, is not the case. As Dr Salen pointed out, given a mixture of CDCA and UDCA, the deleterious effects - if one can put it that way - of UDCA alone in solubilizing biliary cholesterol are very much minimized. There were further details in Dr Carey's letter about total lipid concentration and about the molar ratios of bile acid : phospholipid which are neither appropriate for today's discussion, nor are they likely to be of major importance in the fairly narrow range of variation found in the clinical setting.

Grundy: We really do not know all the reasons why CDCA works better than cholate; the physical chemical data do not suggest that CDCA dissolves stones better than cholate; therefore other factors must be involved. I think that there may be other effects of UDCA or CDCA besides the effects on the solubilization of cholesterol in bile, i.e. physiological effects, and these have not been worked out at all yet. They may be more important in explaining the solubilization of gallstones than the physical chemistry.

Stiehl: I learned from Professor Dowling's work that all the people who did not respond to CDCA did not respond with their cholesterol saturation index. I am therefore surprised to hear that the cholesterol saturation index may not be as important as we thought.

What is your personal opinion of this somewhat conflicting situation?

Dowling: I do not think we are being quoted quite correctly.

Stiehl: You told us that the patients who did not dissolve their gallstones were those who did not drop their cholesterol saturation index sufficiently. The cholesterol saturation index should be of some importance for the clinic, too. Yet we now learn that cholesterol saturation may not in fact be as important as we thought, and I should like to hear an opinion about this.

Dowling: We have no reason to change our opinion on the basis of our studies with UDCA. That is not to say that there is 100% black and white separation between the responders whose stones dissolve and the non-responders whose X-rays show no change, because biomedical science does not work that way. By and large, we find that the saturation index is a useful predictor. At the same time we should stress that it is not necessary to monitor the bile lipid response to treatment in all patients since this is not really practical. But if we are measuring the saturation index in UDCA-treated patients, I do not think that the correction factor we need to apply is *likely* to be of any major importance.

Salen: About the cholesterol saturation index, it is important to note that it is measured on samples of duodenal bile during the administration of bile acids. I wonder whether more impressive values would be obtained if the saturation index could be measured in samples of hepatic bile. Bile is secreted by the liver and enters the gallbladder where we hope it will take up additional cholesterol from the gallstones. Actually, we hope that this bile becomes fully saturated with cholesterol from the gallstones, so that looking at the duodenal saturation index may not be accurate. As a matter of fact, the more unsaturated the duodenal bile, the slower the gallstones may dissolve.

Hofmann: This is a crucial point. When we began our studies with CDCA at the Mayo Clinic, and these were largely carried out by J. L. Thistle and L. J. Schoenfield (1971), we reasoned that if the stones would have equilibrated with bile, they would have disappeared in 2 weeks and fasting-state bile would have remained saturated, being filled with cholesterol from the dissolving gallstones. As Dr Fromm stated, in agreement with our collaborative studies with Dr Higuchi at the University of Michigan (Kwan *et al.*, 1977), when lecithin is present with bile acids, cholesterol dissolves very slowly. I do not think that we can prove this point, but my guess is that the saturation increase induced by gallstone dissolution is too small to measure. Indeed, it must be because not more than 1-3 mg/day of a gallstone is dissolved during chenotherapy, and this is less than 0.1% of daily biliary cholesterol secretion.

The point that I wanted to make about saturation is that we cannot confidently assume that every patient's bile falls exactly on the Hegardt-Dam-Holzbach line. We have tested this assumption experimentally in relatively few patients. It is an assumption, and it is probably correct; but we should label it an assumption. It would not hurt to have a little bit more experimental confirmation.

Dowling: Dr Salen is stimulating us all by playing the role of *agent provocateur*. He made a comment earlier, to which no one replied, about the mechanism of action of UDCA and the assumption that when there is a lot of UDCA in the intestine, it may inhibit cholesterol solubility and absorption. Does anyone want to discuss this?

Hofmann: Together with Dr Thistle, Dr Tangedahl and Dr Matseshe (1977), we measured the effect of CDCA on cholesterol absorption using the isotope ratio technique. We found no effect, in agreement with the earlier work of Adler and Grundy (1975). When we gave β-sitosterol, we clearly abolished the absorption of cholesterol, yet the effect of bile saturation was extremely small.

I therefore think that Dr Salen is correct in raising the point that we do not know whether UDCA will influence cholesterol absorption. However, in my opinion, even if it does, this effect is not likely to have a very important effect on bile saturation. That is an opinion, and I have no experimental evidence.

Dowling: In terms of the effects of different UDCA doses and UDCA-CDCA comparisons, I should like to turn now to the evidence from dose-response studies, dealing first with bile lipids and then with the effect of UDCA therapy on biliary bile acid composition.

Thistle: We fed doses of UDCA and CDCA of approximately 5 and 10 mg/kg-day, prescribed in random order during four consecutive periods of 6 weeks each to each of six men. All of these patients had multiple radiolucent gallstones in well visualizing gallbladders and bile supersaturated with cholesterol. After treatment with both the low and moderate doses of UDCA, bile became unsaturated in five of the six patients. In contrast, with identical doses of CDCA in the same patients, bile became unsaturated in only one of the six. This comparison is based on the assumption that the Hegardt-Dam line (1971) is appropriate to use when the UDCA content of bile is increased. The validity of this has yet to be established. In summary, we found very distinct differences between the effects of UDCA and CDCA on bile saturation in this small number of patients (Thistle *et al.*, 1978).

Fromm: I am sure that Dr Thistle mentioned this, but for how many days?

Thistle: Six weeks for each one. Twenty-four weeks per patient.

Salen: I have a general question. Can we predict from the oral dose how much bile acid enters the pool, especially since bacteria degrade CDCA and UDCA to some extent?

Dowling: The point is obviously interesting, but is it relevant to dose response in measuring bile lipids?

Salen: Surely it is relevant. How can there be a dose response if one does not know the dose?

Thistle: I believe the usual interpretation of the word 'dose', when applied to a dose response study, refers to the orally-ingested dose. The physiological effect is dependent on a number of factors. This is also the way we approach treatment of patients, i.e. the dose ingested is related to the physiological effect. The multifactorial mechanism for that effect is somewhat of another matter and relates to a number of variables, including bioavailability.

Hofmann: Let us be very clear on one thing. Even if we disagree, let us be clear. Both CDCA and UDCA are probably fully bioavailable; thus, one absorbs what one ingests. The bile acid is absorbed as the unconjugated bile acid without dehydroxylation in the small intestine. Dehydroxylation does not occur until each molecule has made multiple trips in the enterohepatic circulation. This is true both for CDCA and UDCA, or at least that is what I believe.

Salen: I do not think so at all. I bring this question up because I have trouble understanding some of the responses. I do not question, but I bring up these possibilities.

We feed the bile acid in divided doses during the day, but we sample the bile one time, generally fasting, the following morning. That will obviously affect the interpretation of the experiment. What we should like to know is the continuous bile saturation data. If the CDCA was completely absorbed, we would expect to see comparable levels of desaturation immediately after the CDCA was ingested. However, we are actually sampling the bile after the bile acid has entered the enterohepatic circulation and circulated for at least 12-24 hours.

Dowling: Dr Salen is asking for data which we do not have - unless Dr Grundy has information about this based on secretion/perfusion studies?

Grundy: No, but Dr Salen has a point that the composition of the bile acid pool is not simply a function of the first-pass clearance, but is an accumulative effect.

Hofmann: Yes. But the dose absorbed in each oral dose, if the patient takes 250 mg q.i.d., is quite small compared to normal bile acid secretion (6000-12000 mg/day). Thus, my view, which may not be right, is that the effect of that acute dose on bile saturation is really negligible.

In other words, if the patient were to stop taking the CDCA for 3 days, and if bile saturation was measured each day, bile would resaturate only extremely slowly (Iser *et al.*, 1977).

Salen: The question about the different rate of bacterial metabolism of CDCA and UDCA and lithocholate formation might be relevant to this part. Further, I know of no studies as yet where people have compared the effect of bile acid feeding and biliary lipid composition, with time.

Dowling: Professor Dioguardi and Dr Podda have also done some work in this field.

Podda: We have given UDCA to ten patients. The mean dose was 7.8 mg/kg-day with a range of 6.8-8.5 mg/kg-day for a mean period of 40 days with a range of 33-48 days. We sampled bile and determined its lithogenic index calculated according to Hegardt and Dam (1971) in 22 patients with cholesterol gallstones and functioning gallbladders. The mean lithogenic index before treatment was 1.37, and it was 0.73 after treatment. Only in three patients did UDCA fail to reduce the saturation index below 1.0. Of those three patients, one was a diabetic, and a second had gallstones in the bile duct.

When UDCA was administered at the same dose in the same patients over the same period of treatment, the lithocholic acid was unchanged, the proportion of cholic, deoxycholic, and chenodeoxycholic acids fell significantly and the UDCA increased from 2 to 39%.

35

We found a very significant correlation between the lithogenic index and the percentage of UDCA in biliary bile acid, as well as between the lithogenic index and UDCA plus the CDCA. But even more significant, these data were obtained during treatment and after 40 days of treatment without taking basal rates into account. If basal values were added in, then the correlation index was even more significant.

Dowling: By basal values you mean that you have included the pre-treatment values with the on-treatment values?

Podda: Yes. The correlation coefficient was −0.81 for UDCA alone, and −0.87 between the lithogenic index and UDCA plus CDCA.

Dowling: These are interesting results, but you have told us mainly about single UDCA doses and not about the effect of different doses.

Stiehl: We studied 20 patients on 10 mg/kg and 10 patients on 15 mg/kg UDCA. We can confirm that the saturation index decreases with increasing UDCA dose. When we analyzed the bile at the higher dose, we found higher concentrations of UDCA in bile, and with these higher concentrations of UDCA in bile, we found lower cholesterol saturation indices. We can therefore be pretty sure that the higher the dose, the more UDCA appears in the bile, and the greater the degree of desaturation.

In some patients, at a dose of 15 mg/kg, we observed cholesterol saturation indices of 0.4, a degree of desaturation we never achieved during CDCA treatment (Stiehl *et al.*, 1978).

Dowling: Dr Thistle showed that at around 5 mg UDCA per kg-day that some patients still had supersaturated bile, even though the mean saturation index was significantly different from the pre-treatment period. We must think in terms of a dose which will not only produce a statistically significant change, but one which will be effective in the majority of patients.

Roda, A.: Our investigations were carried out to study the effect of short term administration of high doses of UDCA on the biliary bile acid pattern, evaluated by gas/liquid chromatography (Roda, A. *et al.*, in press) as well as fasting-state biliary lipid composition (saturation index) (Hegardt and Dam, 1971). Seven patients (five women and two men, mean age 44 years) with cholesterol gallstones in functioning gallbladders were studied. UDCA was administered at a dose of 12 mg/kg-day. Patients were not receiving any other drugs. None were overweight. UDCA

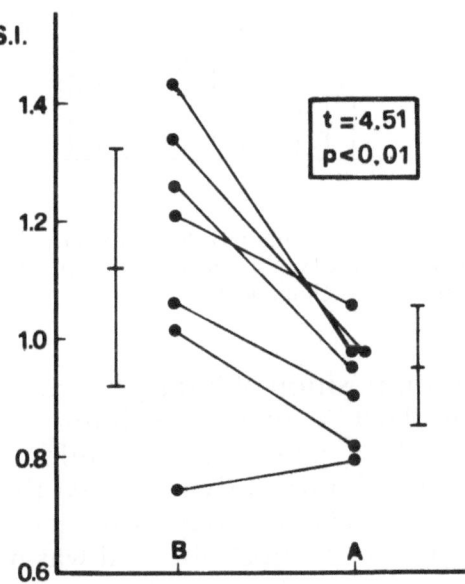

Figure 7 Saturation index (SI) before (B) and 1 month after (A) UDCA treatment (12 mg/kg-day) (Mean ± SD)

administration improved cholesterol solubility (Figure 7). The saturation index fell significantly ($p < 0.01$) passing from 1.16 ± 0.2 (M $\pm$ SD) to 0.93 ± 0.14. In all but one patient, bile became unsaturated in cholesterol.

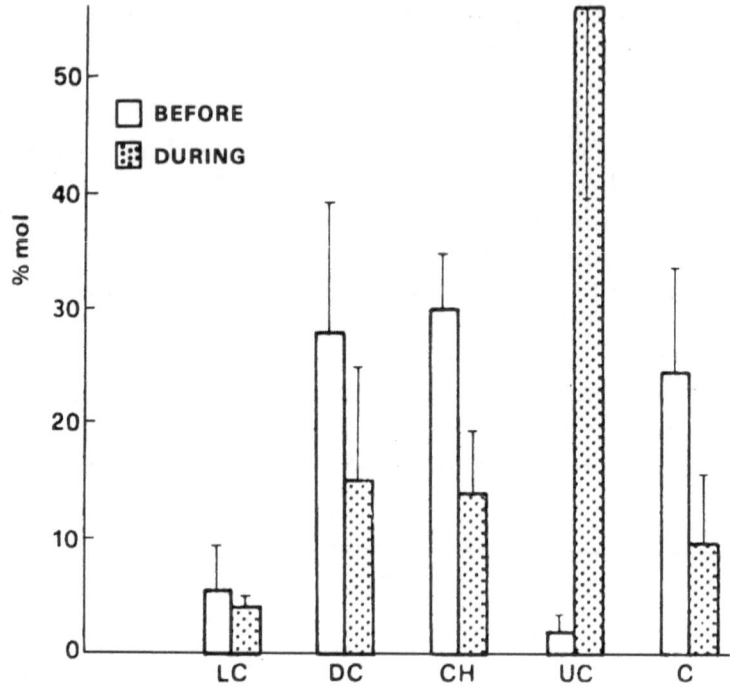

Figure 8 Biliary bile acid patterns before and during UDCA therapy. LC = lithocholic acid; DC = deoxycholic acid; CH = chenodeoxycholic acid; UC = ursodeoxycholic acid; C = cholic acid

Per cent composition of biliary bile acids was markedly affected by UDCA therapy (Figure 8), with UDCA becoming the predominant bile acid. UDCA administration significantly decreased the proportion of cholic acid ($p < 0.005$), deoxycholic acid ($p < 0.01$), and CDCA ($p < 0.001$). Lithocholic acid was not significantly affected.

Grundy: What proportion of bile acids became UDCA? Did you measure that?

Podda: At 12 mg/kg UDCA composed about 50% of biliary bile acids.

Grundy: The per cent of UDCA does not go up as much as CDCA for a given dose, does it? That could be important.

Dowling: Can you confirm that despite treatment with 12 mg UDCA per kg, some of your patients were left with supersaturated bile - is that correct? That is a somewhat different pattern of response from what others are finding.

Hofmann: What is the percentage of patients who did not desaturate?

Roda, A.: In our cases, in six patients the bile desaturated, and in one it did not.

Miettinen: Is the change in cholesterol saturation dependent on the obesity of the subject?

Roda, A.: The group was of normal weight.

Hofmann: We are in a new area of medical research, and we are really all trying to find the best kinds of experiments to do. It is important to compare CDCA against UDCA in the same patients.

Professor Dowling has recently documented biological resistance to CDCA. It seems important to find out whether some patients who respond to CDCA do not respond to UDCA, or vice versa. I do not think it likely, but we may well have to do crossover studies to find out.

Dowling: The studies on biological resistance to CDCA to which you refer were carried out by Dr Maton, and he will be discussing them later.

Salen: I have no wish to be disagreeable, but I should like to bring up the point about the comparison. When we feed CDCA, we get some UDCA in the bile, and when we feed UDCA, we get CDCA in the bile.

I should like to suggest that we look at the two together in making the comparison. It might give us a more meaningful insight into what is happening.

Dowling: That is obviously one way of approaching the problem, but if you are agreeable, we might defer discussion about CDCA-UDCA comparisons until later.

Gasbarrini: We have some data concerning the lithogenic index (LI) of bile in three groups of patients: hyperlipemic without gallstones, hyperlipemic with gallstones, and patients with gallstones only. Patients were given UDCA in doses of 10 mg/kg body weight per day. All patients adhered to their usual diet. The lithogenic index was calculated after 2, 4, and in two cases, 8 weeks of treatment.

We have not done any statistical evaluation of our data because they need further investigations. Nearly all the hyperlipemic subjects with or without gallstones had unsaturated bile before UDCA treatment and the LI was not changed during the first 4-week period of therapy; in one patient, however, the LI was more than 1 and fell to less than 0.2 after 2 weeks of treatment. In a patient with type V hyperlipemia, the LI was 2.2 before UDCA and 1.7 after 2 weeks of treatment.

Another patient suffering from hyperlipemia and cholesterol gallstones had a LI of 0.8 in basal conditions and 0.4 after 2 weeks of UDCA. In this patient the interruption of the treatment resulted in a rise in the LI to 1.2 during the first 2 weeks.

Dowling: Two comments. First, I am very pleased to see that you are looking at the speed of change in bile composition with time after starting therapy, but some of us are surprised that before treatment six of your eight patients had unsaturated bile and some of them had saturation indices of 0.2-0.3, which is very different from what the majority of other investigators find. Can you explain?

Gasbarrini: They are hyperlipemic subjects without gallstones.

Dowling: Even so, it is still strange.

Gasbarrini: I think that changes in LI may occur in the same subject. Our opinion is that there is a great variability in the LI of hyperlipemic patients if they do not have gallstones. In our opinion, it is of some interest that no changes occurred in the LI during UDCA treatment when the LI ranged between 0.2 and 0.4 in patients with hyperlipemia with or without gallstones.

Dowling: What kind of hyperlipemic patients? Was it mixed hyperlipidemia, hypercholesterolemia, hyper-triglyceridemia, or was it type IV?

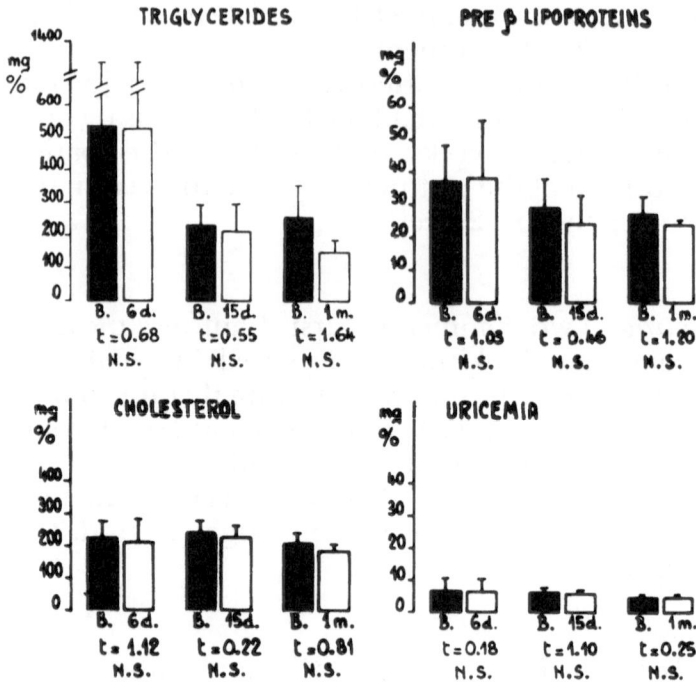

Figure 9 Effect of CDCA treatment on serum levels of triglycerides, pre-ß-lipoproteins (upper panels), cholesterol, and uric acid (lower panels) for 6 days (left), 15 days (centre), and 1 month (right)

Gasbarrini: They were all type IV, except one which was type V.

In these patients we have also carried out a study on serum lipid changes after 6, 15, and 30 days of treatment; serum triglycerides and pre-ß-lipoproteins fell after UDCA therapy, but the differences were not statistically significant (Figure 9, with B = base; d = day; m = month).

Salvioli: Even in my experience, the SI was sometimes greater than 1.0 after 6-8 weeks of UDCA therapy. I have treated, to date, 11 patients with doses of UDCA ranging from 6.9-15 mg/kg-day. The results were analyzed according to multiple regression analysis: the SI after treatment fell in all cases and was significantly correlated with only the pre-treatment values (Figure 10).

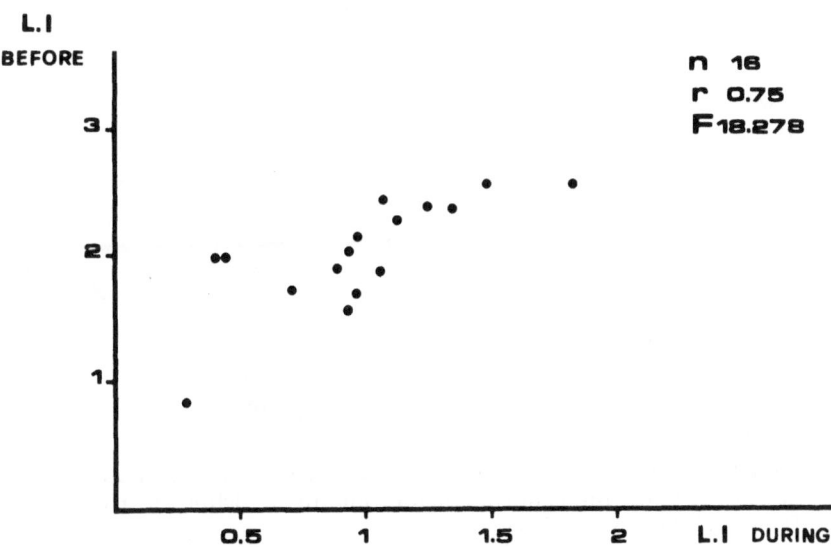

Figure 10 Relationship between saturation index of fasting-state duodenal bile before (ordinate) and during (abscissa) treatment with UDCA in gallstone patients. The effect on the saturation of bile is already present at the minimum doses employed

Maton: For our study (Maton *et al.*, 1977), we took 11 non-obese patients all with radiolucent stones in a functioning gallbladder. Each patient took three doses of UDCA - 6 weeks treatment with approximately 5 mg/kg-day, followed by 6 weeks at 10 mg/kg-day, and then 6 weeks at 15 mg/kg-day. Duodenal intubation was carried out to obtain bile-rich duodenal juice for determination of fasting-state biliary lipids before treatment and at the end of each 6-week period. Figure 11 shows the relationship between saturation index (using the criteria of Hegardt and Dam, 1971) and the dose of CDCA in mg/kg-day. There was a significant correlation between these variables, with a progressive fall in saturation index as the dosage increased.

Proportions of biliary bile acids after the 5, 10 and 15 mg doses are shown in Figure 12. I should like to make two points from the figure. First, the percentage of UDCA in bile increased progressively with each dose, but did not

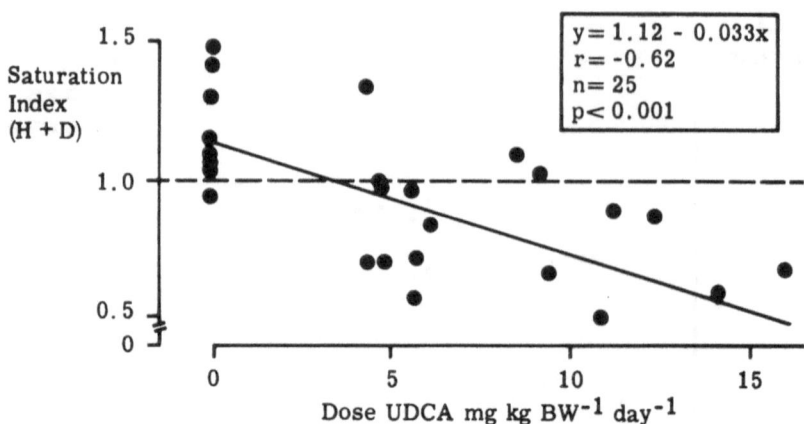

Figure 11 Relationship between biliary cholesterol saturation index (according to the limits of cholesterol solubility as defined by Hegardt and Dam) and the dose of UCDA

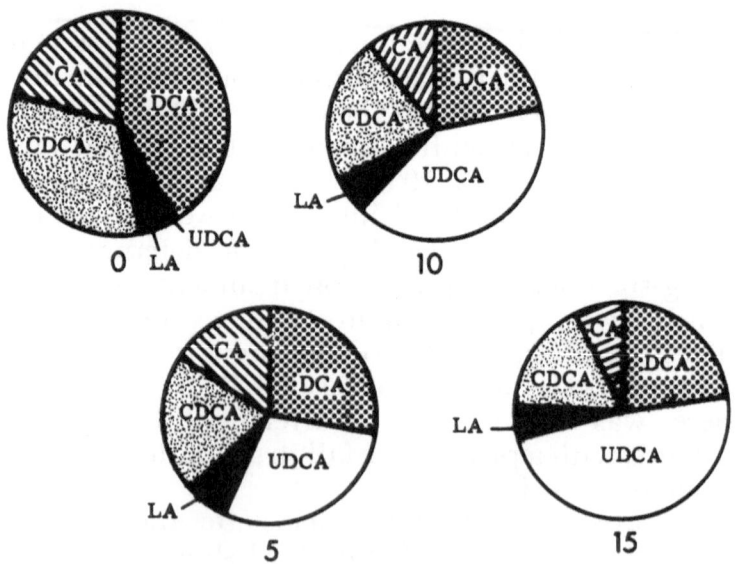

Figure 12 Proportions of biliary bile acids in bile before treatment and on different doses of UDCA (in mg/kg-day)

44

exceed 50%, and secondly, the proportion of lithocholic acid did not significantly increase on UDCA treatment.

Figure 13 shows the relationship between saturation index and the percentage UDCA conjugates in biliary bile acids in the upper panel and UDCA plus CDCA in the lower panel. In both cases, there was a significant correlation.

Fromm: We have also observed a consistent increase in the percentage of UDCA in bile with increasing doses of UDCA. The highest percentage that we recorded was 65% at a dose of about 11 mg/kg body weight -

Dowling: - which is obviously very different from the percentages that are found when CDCA is fed, after which the chenodeoxycholate conjugates in biliary bile acids approach 75-90%.

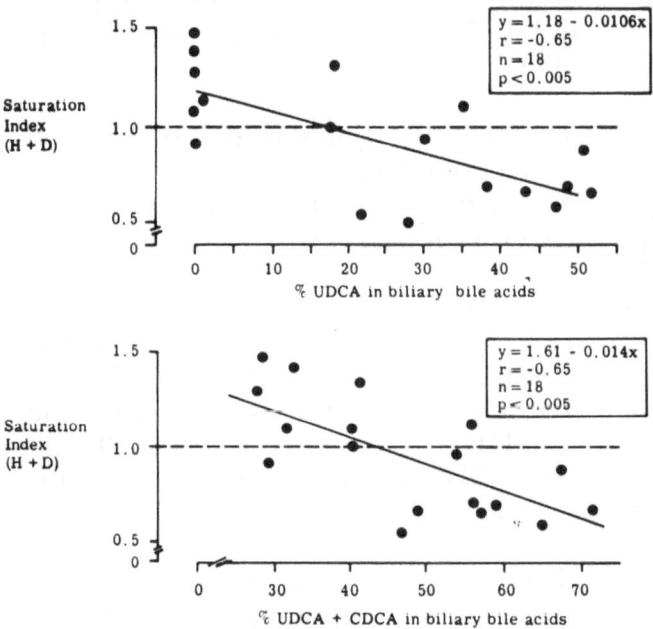

Figure 13 Relationship between biliary cholesterol saturation index and percentage UDCA (upper panel) and UDCA + CDCA (lower panel) in biliary bile acids

Grundy: Can we conclude that UDCA does not inhibit bile acid synthesis?

Hofmann: Dr Thistle has some fecal bile acid data that appear to support this. It is likely that CDCA turns off its own synthesis. We know it turns off cholic acid synthesis (Danzinger *et al.*, 1972). It is likely that UDCA does not suppress CDCA synthesis.

The second effect is, as Dr Salen has shown, that the UDCA is in part converted to CDCA (Fedorowski *et al.*, 1977). I believe that these are two important effects. Although Dr Salen said that there is an increase in UDCA in people taking CDCA, the data from the Mayo Clinic is that this effect is very minor. Most people taking CDCA, and Professor Dowling's data agree, do not get more than 3-4% UDCA in bile (Hofmann *et al.*, 1978).

Thistle: Actually, if one combines the total percentage of CDCA and UDCA, one will come up to 80-90% with feeding UDCA.

Dowling: Dr Grundy's point is an important one - the differential effect of different bile acids on synthesis rates. Perhaps we can get some information about this from fecal bile acid excretion patterns?

Thistle: Biliary bile acid data following treatment with high and low dose UDCA and CDCA demonstrated changes as might be expected from the treatment. The ingested bile acid became the predominant bile acid in bile, although UDCA became only 40 and 50% of total bile acids, whereas CDCA became 75 and 80%. Only 2-3% lithocholate was present after each of the treatment periods.

The fecal bile acid composition after 10 mg/kg-day of the two bile acids was different only with regard to a significantly higher proportion of deoxycholate after UDCA, consistent with the higher biliary proportion of cholic and deoxycholic acids.

Hofmann: That is consistent with UDCA not turning off cholic acid synthesis, because there is more deoxy, assuming that all other factors are equal.

Grundy: If the deoxycholate plus cholate are added together, then it is about 25% which could be equivalent to a synthesis of about 250 mg/day, which is what a person normally makes.

Dowling: Has anybody information about another index of bile acid synthesis - cholesterol 7α-hydroxylase activity in liver biopsies?

Hofmann: We shall hear about this later. Has anybody found 3α-7-keto in bile or feces?

Roda, A: We identified fecal bile acids using a gas/liquid chromatographic method (Grundy *et al.*, 1965; Roda, A.

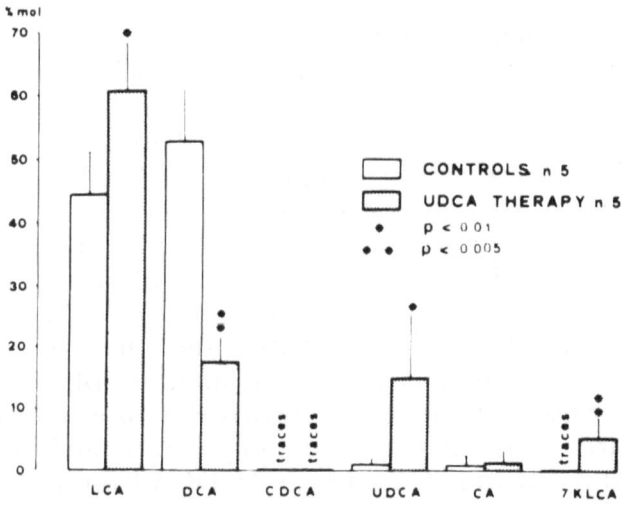

Figure 14 Fecal bile acid composition after 3 months of ursodeoxycholic acid therapy (dose 12 mg/kg-day) (Mean ± SD). LCA = lithocholic acid; DCA = deoxycholic acid; CDCA = chenodeoxycholic acid; UDCA = ursodeoxycholic acid; CA = cholic acid; 7KLCA = 7-ketolithocholic acid

et al., 1977a) in five control subjects and five patients receiving UDCA (dose 12 mg/kg-day). After UDCA, the fecal bile acid pattern changed markedly (Figure 14). Lithocholic acid increased significantly, deoxycholic acid fell, CDCA and cholic acid did not increase, and UDCA was present in 15% of total bile acids. In addition, we found a detectable amount of 7-keto-lithocholic acid (5% of total bile acids); these patients did not have diarrhea. Therefore, these data suggest that (a) UDCA does not induce diarrhea (CDCA at the same percentage in feces induces diarrhea), and (b) a possibility of interconversion of UDCA into CDCA via 7-keto-lithocholic acid.

Dowling: Earlier, there was a question about whether or not UDCA has a lesser effect in inhibiting bile acid synthesis than CDCA. Has anybody carried out isotope dilution studies to obtain information about synthesis rate?

Mazzella: Primary bile acids and total bile acid pool sizes had been evaluated in seven patients before and 1 month after the beginning of UDCA treatment (12 mg/kg-day), according to Lindstedt's method (Lindstedt, 1957) after intravenous injection of 5 μCi of 24-^{14}C-CDCA. In five of the same patients, the turnover of cholic acid was also studied simultaneously after intravenous injection of 10 μCi of 2,4-^{3}H-cholic acid (LaRusso *et al.*, 1974). Cholic acid pool and total bile acid pool were calculated from the measured CDCA pool and the bile acid composition in bile, assessed by gas/liquid chromatography.

We observed a decrease in primary bile acid pool sizes (Figure 15); namely, cholic acid passed from 554 ± 300 mg to 185 ± 137 mg ($p < 0.01$) and CDCA from 738 ± 203 mg to 168 ± 104 mg ($p < 0.001$). The cholic and CDCA turnovers (K) increased significantly, passing from 0.26 ± 0.08 to 1.42 ± 0.83 ($p < 0.001$) and 0.24 ± 0.09 to 0.71 ± 0.26 ($p < 0.005$), respectively. Cholic acid synthesis seemed not to be affected by UDCA administration while CDCA synthesis appeared decreased by 36%. However, this is not statistically significant. In two patients, in fact, CDCA synthesis was augmented, perhaps due to the conversion

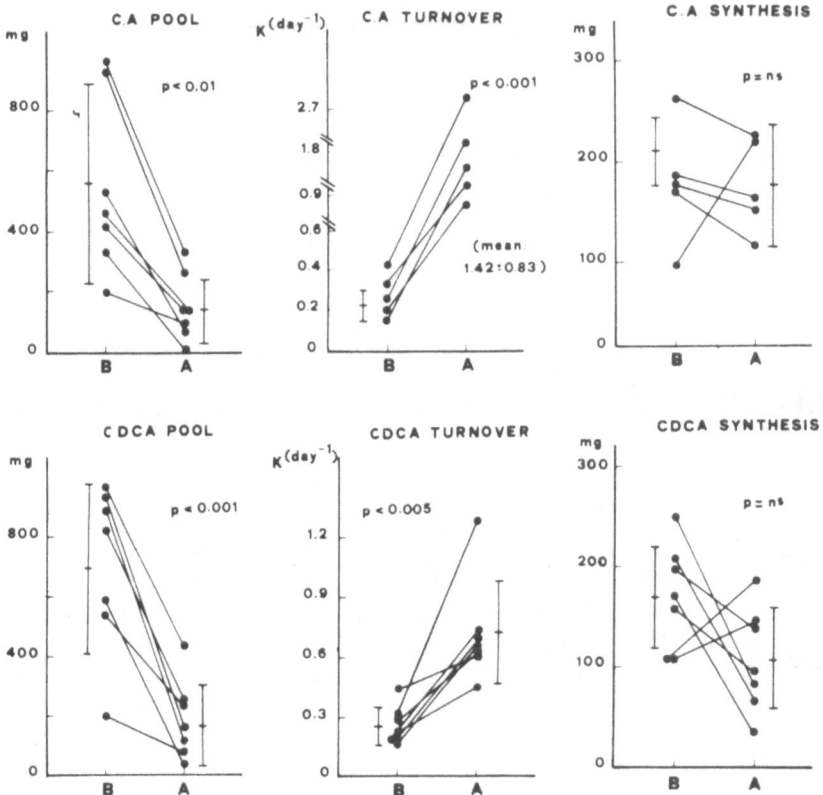

Figure 15 Pool size, fractional turnover rate, and daily synthesis rate of primary bile acids before (B) and after (A) ursodeoxycholic acid therapy. CA = cholic acid; CDCA = chenodeoxycholic acid

of UDCA to CDCA. Total bile acid pool (Figure 16) decreased, passing from 2228 ± 337 mg to 1317 ± 469 mg after 1 month of UDCA therapy. The result is statistically significant ($p < 0.005$).

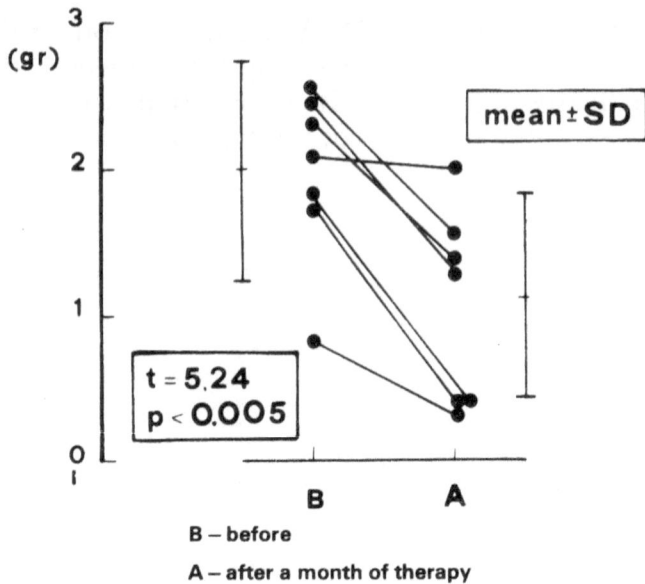

Figure 16 Total bile acid pool before (B) and after (A) UCDA treatment for 1 month

Hofmann: To my knowledge, there are no data on the effect of UDCA on CDCA synthesis. The previous figure suggests that UDCA inhibits CDCA synthesis, but not that of cholic. That is very fascinating. If true, it is the first example of specificity in the negative feedback regulation of bile acid synthesis. It agrees with the fecal bile acid data that UDCA has an effect on CDCA synthesis, but not on that of cholic.

Dowling: When you say the 'first example', there is the much debated evidence from the Bristol group that deoxycholic acid has a selective effect on the synthesis of CDCA (Low-Beer and Pomare, 1975), but these findings conflict with the results of studies from your own Unit (LaRusso *et al.*, 1977) and with the findings of the Swedish group (Einarsson *et al.*, 1974).

Hofmann: Our studies and the Swedish studies show no specific effect. Deoxycholic acid administration caused inhibition of both cholic and CDCA synthesis. I realize these studies disagree with the earlier report of Low-Beer and Pomare (1975), and I do not have an explanation for this disagreement.

Dowling: I was just making the point about your statement that it was the 'first example'.

Hofmann: I am sorry; I was incorrect.

Salen: I should like to comment briefly. In our studies, which we have reported in part at this meeting, where we fed unlabeled UDCA, and then 2 weeks later pulse-labeled the individual with radioactive UDCA, we detected radioactive CDCA. We showed a precursor-product relationship between the radioactive CDCA curve and the radioactive UDCA curve. This means that the CDCA that was present in our patients must have originated from the UDCA, and that, therefore, no endogenous synthesis of the CDCA occurred. UDCA seems to have a selective effect in inhibiting CDCA synthesis, but apparently not cholic acid synthesis.

Mazzella: I agree.

Hofmann: What one obtains using the isotope dilution technique is the input of unlabeled CDCA from two sources - either biotransformation of UDCA or synthesis from cholesterol. These cannot be distinguished. Therefore, if the input of CDCA diminishes, it means that the effect of UDCA on its synthesis may be especially marked.

Dowling: Has anyone carried out isotope dilution studies of this sort in the same individuals who were first given CDCA and then UDCA?

(No response).

Hofmann: To answer Dr Grundy's point, we cannot validly compare two separate groups. We should look at synthesis rates in the same individual during sequential treatments with CDCA and UDCA. The experiment probably has to be done by labeling the cholesterol pool. Although many people talk about the experiment, no one has done it yet. However, I believe that Dr Quarfordt is doing it at the moment.

Chadwick: May I ask the Bologna group about the interesting effect on turnover, suggesting that UDCA is interfering with bile acid absorption? Can we explain the changes in turnover of the bile acids during UDCA therapy? It suggests an interference with absorption. We were told that the effects on synthesis rate were not significant, but I agree with Professor Hofmann that it looks as though there was something in it.

Mazzella: The measured turnover suggests that UDCA may interfere with the absorption of the primary bile acids, but I have not studied the problem.

Hofmann: That is right. Any time when one feeds a bile acid, one increases the turnover of the other bile acids, because they compete for active absorption. I think that is completely reasonable.

Grundy: Is it really true that the total bile acid pool is reduced during feeding of UDCA? How did you make the measurement? I misunderstood the method of measuring total bile acids. What did you use? What isotopes did you use?

Mazzella: We have used the Lindstedt method (1957), 24-^{14}C-CDCA and 2,4-^{3}H-cholic acid were used as tracers. Cholic acid pool and total bile acid pool were calculated from the measured CDCA pool and from the bile acid composition of bile, assessed by gas/liquid chromatography.

Grundy: Does this total pool include UDCA?

Mazzella: Yes.

Grundy: So you think the total pool is reduced? It is astonishing.

Hofmann: But it is known that the pool may go down in patients taking CDCA, too. We found such patients (Danzinger *et al.*, 1972), and I believe that Dr Fromm found such patients (Fromm *et al.*, 1976). When patients with large deoxycholic pools receive CDCA, the decline in the deoxy pool may be so great that the bile acid pool actually decreases in size.

Dowling: Are there any comparable data for pool size in control subjects? I am sure that what Professor Hofmann says is true, but, by and large, where there is a small pool before treatment, then after therapy with either cholic or CDCA (as you yourself showed with Rudy Danzinger, 1972) the pool tends to expand and return to normal size.

It would be very nice to know if there are any secretion/perfusion studies to go along with the measurements of bile acid pool and to learn something about what happens to the cycling frequency of the bile acid pool with treatment. One would like to know about the net effect of a reduction in pool size on overall bile acid secretion rates.

Hofmann: There may be an additional problem. As you know, we prepared 11,12-^{3}H-CDCA and 24-^{14}C-CDCA. We lost about 15% of the label from 11,12-^{3}H-CDCA, and accordingly, with this one tends to give a smaller pool size (Ng and Hofmann, 1977).

Mazzella: Yes, I know. 2,4-^{3}H-cholic acid has been used only to measure the turnover rate of cholic acid. In our experience, the turnover of the steroid moieties was the same using either ^{14}C- or ^{3}H-labeled bile acids.

Dowling: If 1 g UDCA is administered per day, how big is the UDCA pool?

Mazzella: The size of the UDCA pool in our patients was 728 ± 301 mg.

Dowling: Since we are talking about synthesis rates, I know that Dr Fromm has a lot of information about intermediary metabolism. Perhaps he can deal with the question that was asked earlier on the formation of 3α-7-keto-cholanoate.

Fromm: The background to our studies was that it is well known that CDCA can be converted to UDCA and UDCA to CDCA. A number of studies in animals (Mahowald *et al.*, 1958; Samuelson, 1959; Hellström and Sjövall, 1960) and also in man (Salen *et al.*, 1974; Hofmann and Paumgartner, 1975; Stiehl *et al.*, 1975; Fromm *et al.*, 1976) clearly showed this.

It has been assumed that 7-keto-lithocholic acid is the intermediate in this conversion reaction, and it has also been shown by other investigators that 7-keto-lithocholic acid can be converted by UDCA and CDCA (Hellström and Sjövall, 1960).

It is of interest to note that 7-keto-lithocholic acid can be present in considerable amounts in the small intestine. Dr Bolt from Chicago has told me that she found considerable amounts of 7-keto-lithocholate in small intestinal contents of a patient with bacterial overgrowth in the small bowel.

7-Keto-lithocholic acid has been found in human feces (Eneroth *et al.*, 1966). In the first study, we investigated the hepatic metabolism of 7-keto-lithocholic acid. An occluding balloon in the second portion of the duodenum was used in order to interrupt the enterohepatic circulation. Tracer amounts of ^{14}C-labeled 7-keto-lithocholic acid, CDCA, and UDCA, respectively, both the free compounds and the conjugates, were injected intravenously. We collected bile proximal to the balloon during continuous intravenous infusion of cholecystokinin.

It was clearly shown that in the liver, the majority of ^{14}C-labeled 7-keto-lithocholic acid was converted to CDCA. A small percentage was converted to UDCA. Some of the label remained unchanged. There were several other metabolites which we did not identify. CDCA and UDCA were not altered during their passage through the liver (Fromm *et al.*, 1977).

In a second study a bolus of 1 mmol ^{14}C-labeled 7-keto-lithocholic acid was infused into the proximal small intestine. Intestinal contents were collected continuously 60 cm distal to the infusion site. In addition, we collected intermittently blood samples for 2 h and bile 1 h after the infusion of the labeled 7-keto-lithocholic acid.

The radioactivity peaked 30 min after the infusion of

7-keto-lithocholic acid. The shape of the radioactivity curve is almost identical to that observed and published by Dr van Berge Henegouwen and Dr Hofmann (1977b), who infused CDCA, indicating that there is good absorption of 7-keto-lithocholic acid.

In addition, we also analyzed the effluent 60 cm distal to the infusion site and found no radioactivity, further indicating that there is good absorption. Gas chromatographic studies of the serum revealed that the radioactivity in the serum represented 7-keto-lithocholic acid (Fromm *et al.*, 1978).

Thin-layer chromatographic bile acid analysis in bile showed the same distribution of the radioactivity we had demonstrated before when we studied one hepatic passage of 7-keto-lithocholic acid.

In summary, the studies indicate that CDCA and UDCA are, probably by intestinal bacteria, oxidized to 7-keto-lithocholic acid which is then reabsorbed and subsequently converted in the liver to CDCA and UDCA.

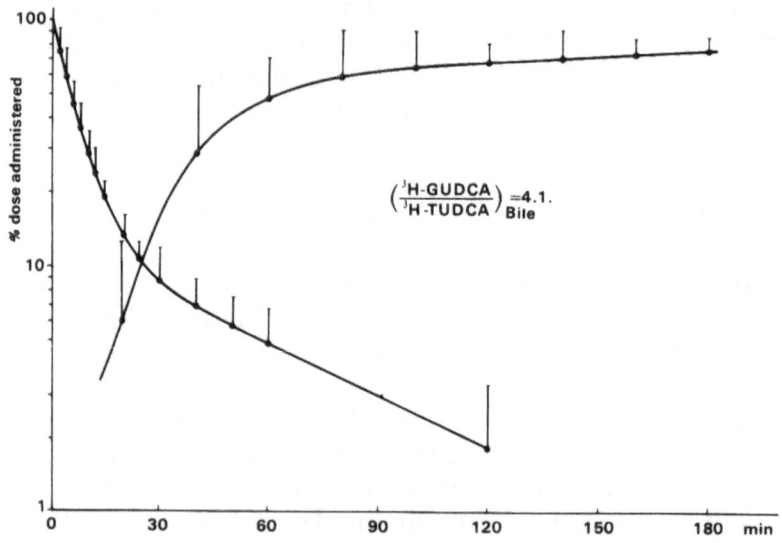

Figure 17 Plasma disappearance and appearance in bile of radioactivity after intravenous injection of ³H-UDCA (30 μCi) in three cholecystectomized patients (Mean ± SD)

Dowling: We have one more piece of information about this interconversion from the Bologna group before we open the matter for more general discussion.

Sama: Figure 17 shows the biotransformation of UDCA after intravenous injection of ^{3}H-labeled UDCA using the same technique with a triple lumen tube with an occludible balloon, as was used by Dr Fromm. We found only conjugates of UDCA in bile, and the glycine : taurine ratio was 4:1. We recovered the majority of the radioactivity after 180 min of collecting bile. We have no experience with 7-keto-lithocholic acid at the moment. We used cholecystectomized patients in order to prevent the effects of gallbladder contraction in the secretion study.

Salen: Although it has been postulated that 7-keto-lithocholic acid serves as an intermediate between the interconversion of CDCA and UDCA and UDCA back to CDCA, I should like to suggest that this pathway is not necessary. The evidence for this was developed when we carried out the experiments incubating intestinal bacteria with radioactive UDCA and radioactive CDCA.

In the experiment with radioactive CDCA, we incubated intestinal bacteria (feces) with radioactive CDCA labeled on the C-24 position. We then carried out this incubation over 24 h, and analyzed incubations hourly for the first 8 h. We isolated the UDCA, CDCA, and the lithocholic acid from the mixtures by thin-layer chromatography, and we measured the amount of radioactivity that was present in each bile acid fraction. Within the first 2 h, radioactive CDCA disappeared very rapidly, associated with a corresponding rise in lithocholic acid. However, of real interest to us was the apparent direct conversion of the CDCA directly to UDCA without 7-keto-lithocholic acid being an intermediate. The mechanism for this reaction was actually suggested by Dr Ferrari (1977) of Milan who has worked in the Institute of Microbiology. The mechanism apparently involves the loss of a water molecule from the CDCA without forming 7-keto-lithocholic acid, but rather the $\Delta^{6,7}$-compound (3α-hydroxy-5β-cholest-6-en-24-oic acid).

I would be happy to discuss the chemistry in more detail if asked.

Hofmann: Can Dr Salen clarify? Has he looked for that $\Delta^{6,7}$-compound?

Salen: We have not looked for the $\Delta^{6,7}$-compound just yet. What must first be done is to synthesize this compound so that we have a reference standard, and we are at work on this problem right now.

Kritchevsky: Is it not possible that there is a small, but rapidly turning over pool of a 7-keto derivative? A pool so small it could not be identified readily?

Salen: That is obviously a possibility, but we would have expected to see 7-keto-lithocholic acid as the UDCA rose over the first 2 h.

Kritchevsky: But this has a parallel in the experiments performed during the elucidation of the pathway of cholesterol biosynthesis. Squalene was unequivocally identified as an intermediate only after that present in liver was trapped by addition of cold squalene prior to workup. Perhaps it would be worthwhile to add the 7-keto compound in hopes that the labeled endogenous intermediate might be trapped.

Salen: We did another experiment to clarify that point. CDCA labeled specifically with ^{3}H in the 7β position was incubated with intestinal bacteria. If the 7-keto-lithocholic acid was an intermediate, then we would find no radioactivity at all in the UDCA that was formed. However, we found the same curve when we used 7β-^{3}H-CDCA as with 24-^{14}C. We are very confident that 7-keto-lithocholic acid is not an intermediate in this transformation.

Dowling: There is time for just two more comments - one from Professor Hofmann, and then we shall leave the last word to Dr Fromm. Your study was done in a test tube with bacteria, while his was carried out *in vivo* where he was actually looking at lithocholate formation and absorption.

Hofmann: I wanted to take the role of Co-chairman and try to integrate the report of Dr Fromm, the report of Dr Salen, and the report of Dr Sama.

First, everybody agrees, so far, that UDCA, when it reaches the liver is conjugated with glycine or taurine and undergoes no further biotransformation.

Second, everybody agrees, I think, that the 3-hydroxy-7-keto compound can be formed in the intestine, probably in the small intestine, and that when it passes through the liver, it is preferentially reduced to CDCA.

Third, Dr Salen has good evidence that UDCA can be converted directly from CDCA. Therefore, UDCA is both a secondary and a tertiary bile acid.

What bothered me, Dr Fromm, and others was this. If the liver reduces the keto compound so preferentially to CDCA, how can we explain the patients, one of which Dr Salen first reported, with 20% UDCA in bile? And Dr Fromm and Dr Stiehl both had patients with very large amounts of UDCA.

It seems to me, therefore, that we have the occasional

patient in whom the CDCA is converted by bacteria to UDCA and that these are those who have very high UDCA in bile.

The only last point I should like to make is that this postulate of the $\Delta^{6,7}$ intermediate is not a new idea. Samuelson showed over 15 years ago (1960) that cholic was converted to deoxycholic by a $\Delta^{6,7}$-intermediate. So it is a common mechanism in the formation of the major secondary bile acids. So I think that everything agrees at the moment.

Fromm: That has been well summarized, but I have one question for Dr Salen. In his studies he has made an observation which suggests that there may be more than one pathway, as Professor Hofmann has mentioned. Has Dr Salen ever incubated 7-keto-lithocholic acid with bacteria to see what the bacteria do to it?

May I make one acknowledgement? Frequently scientists neglect this. This study would not have been possible if Professor Hofmann and Dr Carlson of the Mayo Clinic had not supplied me with some very vital isotopes for these studies.

Dowling: Perhaps we can move on to the clinical aspects of ursotherapy and the efficacy of UDCA treatment. Could we ask Dr Osuga to open the discussion? He has come all the way from Japan for this meeting, and we are very pleased to see him here.

Osuga: For a long time in our country, the bile of the bear has been used as a folk medicine in cases of stomach trouble, biliary colic, or indigestion. As a child, I remember I was given it by my mother. This is a package of such a folk medicine, and it says here the indication, 'stomach trouble or biliary colic, etc.' I know that nowadays real bear bile is extremely valuable and expensive and that someone uses the liver of the fish instead of bear bile, adding the bitter flavor.

So far in our country, there have been two double blind clinical trials using UDCA. One was conducted in Sapporo and was published in a recent *Lancet* (Nakagawa *et al.*, 1977), and the other was conducted in the Tokyo area (Chairman Dr Kameda). We published it only in Japanese (Ashizawa *et al.*, 1977), so today I shall summarize the result of the Tokyo trial very briefly.

The duration of the trial was 6-12 months. The patients with gallstones were divided into three different dose groups. The dose of UDCA was not based on body weight or body surface, but was fixed arbitrarily; one group at 600 mg/day, a second group at 150 mg/day, and a third group on inactive placebo.

The initial number of entry was 151 cases with 72 cases completing the trial. We excluded many cases because of insufficient or inadequate acceptance, and applied strict criteria to the data. All patients had a functioning gallbladder.

Table 2 is the result when we looked at the non-calcified stone cases, with the percentages in parentheses. The efficacy of UDCA - dissolution of stones, or stones diminished in size or in number - was 41% on the 600 mg dose. On the 150 mg dose, it was 18.8%, and it was 6.7% in the placebo group.

Table 2   Efficacy of UDCA: Non-calcified gallstones

	Dissolved	*Diminished*	*No Change*	*Enlarged*	*Total*
UDCA (600 mg/day)	7	3	14	0	24
		10 (41.7)		14 (58.3)	
UDCA (150 mg/day)	2	1	13	0	16
		3 (18.8)		13 (81.2)	
Placebo	1	0	14	0	15
		1 (6.7)		14 (93.3)	
Total	10	4	41	0	55
		14		41	

Percentages in parenthesis

Table 3 Efficacy of UDCA: Non-calcified, floating, and medium size (<15 mm) gallstones

	Dissolved	Diminished	No Change	Enlarged	Total
UDCA (600 mg/day)	3	2	1	0	6
		5 (83.3)		1 (16.7)	
UDCA (150 mg/day)	2	2	4	0	8
		4 (50.0)		4 (50.0)	
Placebo	1	0	5	0	6
		1 (16.7)		5 (83.3)	
Total	6	4	10	0	20
		10		10	

Percentages in parenthesis

Table 3 is the result when we look at the non-calcified, floating and medium-sized stones (< 15 mm in diameter). Although the number of cases is small, the efficacy rises to 83% in the 600 mg/day group. It was less effective, 42.9%, in the 150 mg/day group, and it was much less in the placebo group. The difference between the 600 mg group and the placebo group was statistically significant, and we could find no statistical significance between the 600 mg and 150 mg groups or between the 150 mg and placebo groups. However, we can see the trend toward a dose dependency about the efficacy. But we need to increase the number of patients.

Dowling: It might be helpful to go around the table and hear of other people's experiences about the efficacy of UDCA.

Fromm: Has the dose been calculated on a kilogram body weight basis, as I am sure there are differences in body weight?

Osuga: The average body weight of a Japanese is about 60 kg. So it is about 10 mg/kg body weight. However, in this trial we did not dose on the basis of body weight or body surface. We tried a high dose, a low dose, and a placebo.

Dowling: Dr Fromm's question emphasizes the whole point of whether we should be recommending a fixed dose, irrespective of body weight, or whether we ought to prescribe doses based on body weight.

Stiehl: (On the results of clinical efficacy)

In seven out of 11 patients we have done re-examinations and have found partial dissolution; the stones were smaller in size. In three, the stones were completely dissolved. We gave a dose of 10-15 mg/kg.

Dowling: It would be helpful if, in discussing the results, people would indicate the type of patient treated, the dose of UDCA administered, and the duration of treatment before dissolution and whether it was partial or complete.

Salen: We have analyzed the results of ten patients who were treated with UDCA at 15 mg/kg-day for 1 year. In six of the patients the stones were dissolved, in one partially dissolved, and in three subjects no effect was seen. Another group of ten patients was treated with 250 mg UDCA/day, which is a dose of 3.4 mg/kg-day; we had one person who had the stones dissolve after 6 months.

Maton: Selection of patients is absolutely critical. In a retrospective analysis of our results in patients treated with CDCA (not UDCA), if we take all our 116 patients with radiolucent gallstones in a functioning gallbladder, the per cent efficacy, as judged by partial and complete dissolution, was only 30%. However, in a highly selected group of patients with stones measuring less than 15 mm in diameter, given not less than 13 mg/kg-day CDCA, with unsaturated bile and who had a minimum of 12 months' treatment, then efficacy was 65% complete or 93% partial plus complete. These differences show that before we can assess and compare efficacy figures, precise selection criteria and modes of treatment must be stated.

We are treating 17 patients with UDCA; eight patients have not yet had their first follow-up cholecystogram and three others have had a cholecystectomy. Seven of our patients have completed 6 months' treatment; one patient showed partial gallstone dissolution, five patients still on treatment have shown partial or complete gallstone dissolution, and one patient who went to surgery (because of the development of a non-functioning gallbladder after 6 months' treatment) also showed partial dissolution. Thus, for patients treated for more than 6 months, the efficacy was six out of seven or 87%. Efficacy in patients with small or medium-sized radiolucent stones in a functioning gallbladder who achieve unsaturated bile seems to be similar for both UDCA and CDCA, although I accept that the numbers of patients in the CDCA and UDCA groups are very different. A further caveat is that patients treated with UDCA took a mixed dose, the first 18 weeks of treatment being part of the dose response study, and then they continued on the smallest UDCA dose that had previously produced a saturation index of approximately 0.8 by the Hegardt-Dam criteria (1971).

Fromm: Has Dr Maton data that show a comparison in the dose response between UDCA and CDCA?

Maton: The smallest bile acid dose required to produce unsaturated bile was similar in one group of patients taking CDCA and in a second group taking UDCA - about 4 mg/kg-day. The minimum dosage that consistently produced unsaturated bile and the mean dose that produced a saturation index of approximately 0.8

was about 9.5 mg/kg for UDCA and 14.5 for CDCA. The mean doses required to produce gallstone dissolution, which included the mixed dose regime for UDCA, were 8.0 mg/kg for UDCA and 14.2 mg/kg for CDCA.

Thistle: We have radiological response data on only the six patients participating in our dose comparison study. After the 24-week study period, the stones were completely dissolved in one patient. The stones were smaller in two additional patients, and one patient had a non-opacifying gallbladder. Considering that the bile was unsaturated presumably during less than half of a 24-week treatment period, in most of the patients the radiological response was somewhat astonishing. All patients, however, had multiple small stones which are usually the most susceptible type for dissolution, at least with CDCA.

Salvioli: We treated 31 patients with gallbladder gallstones, and two patients with gallstones in the common duct with doses ranging from 6.9 to 15 mg/kg-day. I have observed, after treatment ranging up to 4 months, six patients with complete dissolution, and seven with partial dissolution. The patients that showed dissolution were treated with doses of 8 mg/kg-day.

Dowling: And of your total of 33 patients, 13 have shown either partial or complete gallstone dissolution, while 20 have shown no response.
   We seem to be getting some sort of a consensus about dose. Efficacy figures are looking very reasonable, and compare at least as well and possibly better than those for CDCA.

Salvioli: Through December, 1977, we treated 31 patients with gallbladder stones, and two with common bile duct stones; we used doses ranging from 6.9 to 15 mg/kg-day. We observed complete dissolution in six patients and partial dissolution in seven patients. In most instances, patients showing dissolution received 8 mg/kg-day UDCA.

Dowling: So it looks as if dissolution occurs at around 8-10 mg/kg-day UDCA.

Gasbarrini: We have only six patients with small or medium-sized radiolucent gallstones, all treated with 10 mg/kg-day for 6 months. One case showed a diminution of gallstone number and size; in two complete dissolution occurred.

Dowling: What do you define as diminution?

Gasbarrini: Diminution means a reduction in size and/or number of the stones of about 50%.

Fromm: How does Dr Dowling define partial dissolution?

Dowling: At this stage in the UDCA story, one has to rely on people giving intermediate results in which somewhat arbitrary definitions have been applied, but ultimately, partial dissolution does not matter if gallstone dissolution never becomes complete. For the moment, we must assume that people are assessing partial dissolution or diminution in gallstone size and number as fairly and as objectively as possible.

Bazzoli: In order to evaluate the efficacy of UDCA in the dissolution of cholesterol gallstones, 60 patients with radiolucent gallstones in functioning gallbladders were randomly allotted to six treatment groups: placebo; CDCA, 15 mg/kg body weight daily; UDCA, 15 mg; UDCA, 10 mg; UDCA, 5 mg; and UDCA, 3 mg. No significant differences were noted among the treatment groups in weight, age and sex distribution. Conventional liver function tests and serum bile acids were determined initially and 3 months thereafter. Patients were questioned about their symptoms before and during treatment. Before treatment and 3 months after initiation of treatment, cholecystograms were performed by a standard method (oral or intravenous drip), and read and compared by radiologists who were not aware of the patients' treatment.

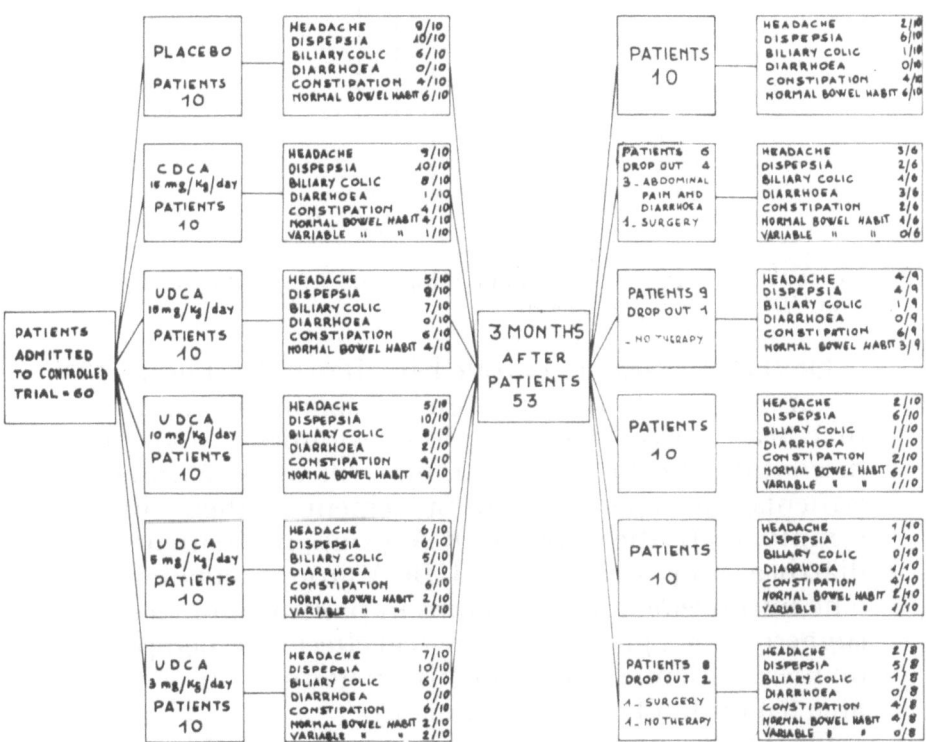

Figure 18   Randomization of patients entered in the UDCA-CDCA-placebo controlled trial and clinical response before and after 3 months of treatment

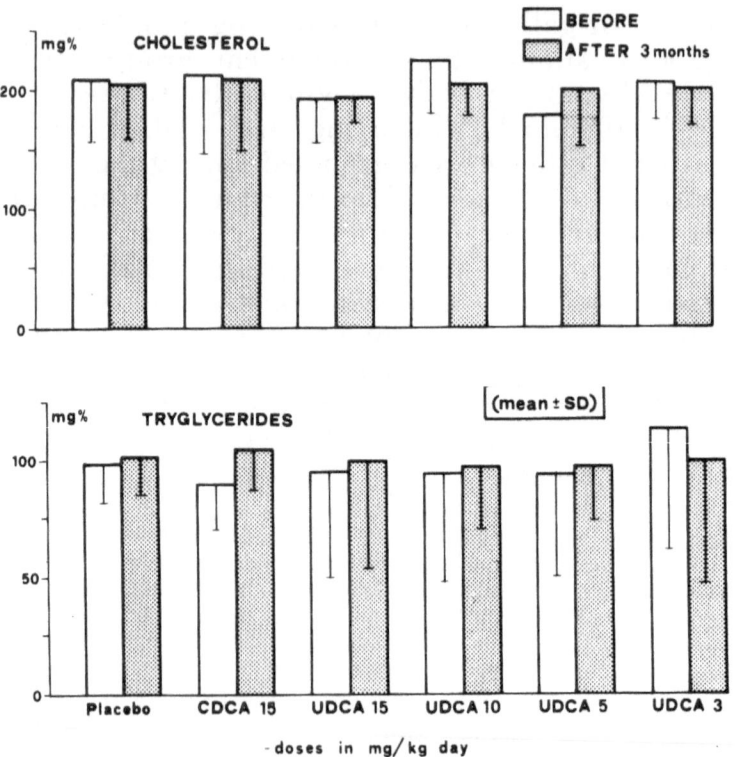

Figure 19 Fasting-state serum lipids before and after 3 months of treatment with UDCA, CDCA, and placebo

Of the 60 patients enrolled in the study (Figure 18), seven dropped out: three due to abdominal pain and diarrhea, two had cholecystectomies, and two discontinued drug administration. Of the remaining 53 patients, all experienced improvement in their clinical symptoms. In the second CDCA group, five patients had diarrhea; no patients in the UDCA groups had diarrhea. The improvement of symptoms in patients on placebo is suggestive of a great psychological effect this therapy had on these patients. The serum lipid pattern was unchanged after 3 months of therapy (Figure 19).

Of the 53 patients remaining in the trial (Figure 20), two were considered inappropriate selections (because the radiologists did not agree on their interpretation of the

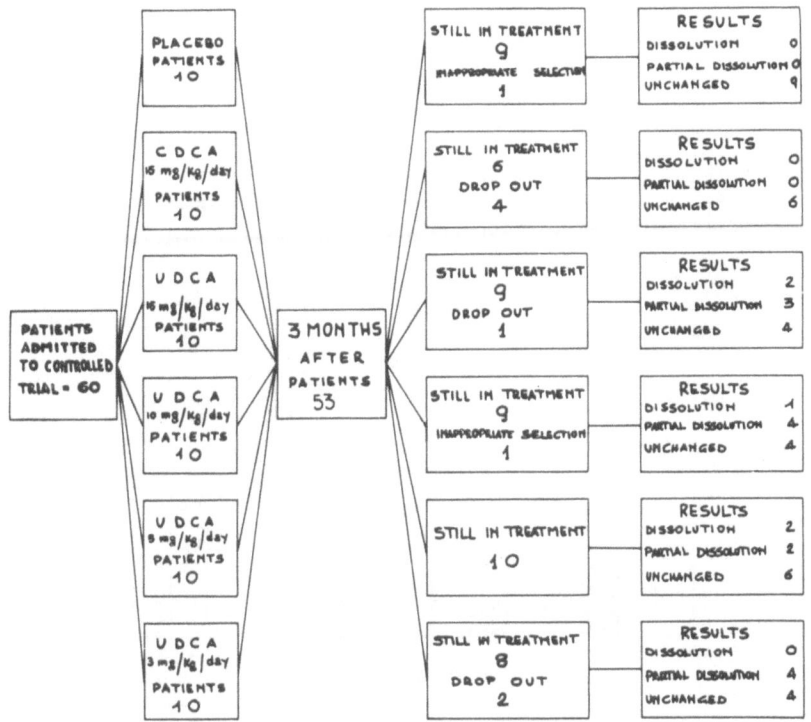

Figure 20 Side effects of UDCA and CDCA in the controlled trial

cholecystograms). No changes were observed in the patients given the placebo and CDCA, 15 mg/kg-day. In patients on UDCA, 15 mg/kg-day, we found two complete dissolutions and three partial dissolutions. In patients on UDCA, 10 mg/kg-day, we found one complete and four partial dissolutions. In patients on UDCA, 5 mg/kg-day, we found two complete and two partial dissolutions. In patients with UDCA, 3 mg/kg-day, we found four partial dissolutions.

Figure 21 summarizes our results in relation to gallstone size. As you can see, we have groups quite homogeneous for size of stones, and we obtained dissolution in patients with stones of different size.

Dowling: That is a wealth of information. The Bologna group has broken many records in this field in the past:

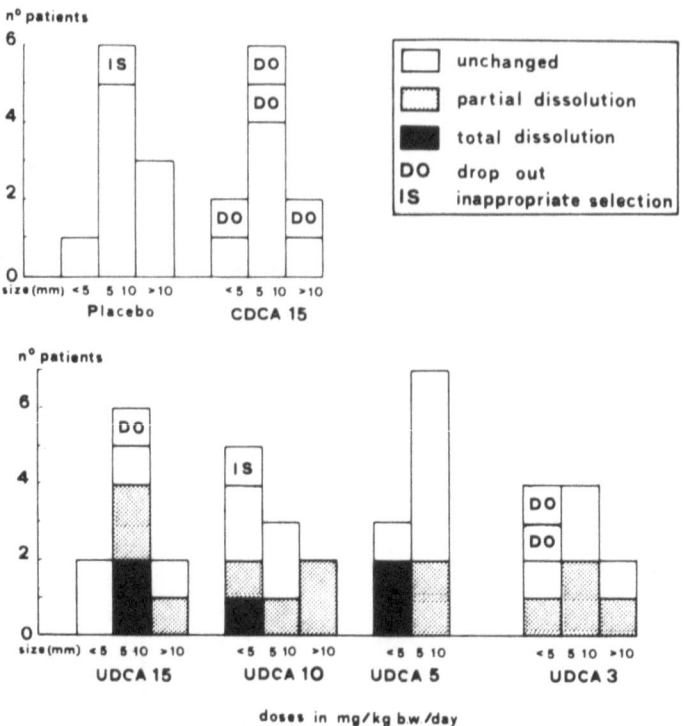

Figure 21 Efficacy of CDCA and UDCA in relation to gallstone size

they have now broken the record for the amount of information contained on a single slide.

Perhaps we should try to summarize all the results on the efficacy of UDCA presented to date. It seems from most studies that UDCA is effective in doses ranging from 8 to 10 mg/kg-day. Would anyone wish to advocate giving a fixed dose, rather than a dose related to body weight? I think the only studies with a fixed dose were those from Dr Osuga in Japan. Is it still your policy to use a fixed dose?

Osuga: We arbitrarily tried the higher dose and the lower doses.

Hofmann: There is a question which is not yet settled. If an excess of CDCA is given, does the bile get still more unsaturated and the stones dissolve rapidly, or is it just wasted? I do not feel that I know the answer to the question. If we would give 10 to 12 mg UDCA/kg, the stone might dissolve more rapidly. Would it cost more for effective treatment to give a higher dose? I do not know the answer. The experiments so far have not answered that question. We clearly have a dose that works well, and I guess the important thing is to err on the side of giving more than is necessary.

Dowling: That is an important point. Dr Fromm has told us that using the largest UDCA dose, he got a saturation index of 0.4. What we do not know is whether stones will dissolve more rapidly or with greater certainty when the saturation index is 0.4 than when it is only 0.8.

Hofmann: To answer that question one would probably have to study at least 100 patients in a double blind study.

We need a lot more information. We shall get this data from the American National Cooperative Gallstone Study. The great problem is that people have different kinds of stones, so to do that, we need to do crossover studies, which may be impossible to do.

Dowling: Some of us around this table are working in University hospitals, but there are also some present who might want practical guidance about the dose and whether they ought to be measuring bile lipids. Therefore, Professor Hofmann's point about fixing a dose which will reliably produce unsaturated bile and dissolve gallstones is really what we need to be aiming for while at the same time keeping costs within reason.

I suggest that we now deal quickly with three topics: (a) diarrhea, (b) the effects of UDCA on the liver, and (c) the mechanism of action of UDCA in desaturating bile and dissolving gallstones.

Has anyone seen diarrhea during ursotherapy, and does anyone have information about the differing effects of UDCA and CDCA on the colon?

Chadwick: I would like to mention data obtained in work carried out together with Sid Phillips and Jean-Claude Debongnie from the Mayo Clinic (Debongnie and Phillips, 1977; Chadwick *et al.*, 1976; Chadwick *et al.*, 1977). The data show the effects of UDCA and CDCA on the perfused human colon. This experiment followed some work in rabbits suggesting that UDCA does not cause secretion in the colon. In this experiment, there is a tube in the distal ileum through which a solution of saline is infused into the cecum at a rate which is related to the normal ileal flow rates - not a fast rate, but a physiological rate. Subsequently, UDCA or CDCA (5 mmol/l sodium salts) is included in the infusate. Fecal weight and fecal sodium output are monitored. It is clear that there is a profound increase in fecal weight and fecal sodium when CDCA was infused, but no difference from control when UDCA was used. These data show that the results that we found in rabbits are also true in man.

Dowling: Has anyone seen diarrhea occurring during UDCA therapy?

Bonvicini: I should like to say something about the correlation between bile acid induced diarrhea and the intracellular levels of cyclic nucleotides.

Previous studies from several laboratories have suggested that cAMP may play a role as mediator in promoting bile acid induced diarrhea (Binder *et al.*, 1975; Conley *et al.*, 1976). With CDCA treatment, we can see that there are parallel increases in both cyclic nucleotides

PATIENTS	DAYS OF CDCA THERAPY (15mg/kg BW/day)	PERCENT INCREASE OF CYCLIC NUCLEOTIDES VERSUS CONTROLS*		NUMBER OF DEFAECATION OF LOOSE STOOLS**
		3'5'AMP	3'5'GMP	
1	5	173.68	266.(6)	7
2	5	152.17	450.00	10
3***	5	172.(2)	125.00	0
4	5	175.00	250.00	10
5***	5	145.00	100.00	0
6	5	183.(3)	333.(3)	11
7	5	139.13	250.00	9
8	10	132.00	225.00	1
9	10	145.00	300.00	3
10	10	117.39	75.00	0
11	10	129.62	180.00	2
12***	10	125.00	100.00	0
13	10	138.09	120.00	1
14	10	132.00	150.00	2
15	15	104.34	160.00	2
16	15	109.52	83.(3)	0
17	15	92.59	100.00	0
18	15	125.00	116.(6)	0
19	15	104.16	160.00	1
20	15	103.84	116.(6)	0
21	15	108.(3)	140.00	0

* CONTROLS EQUAL 100%
** THE EVALUATION REFERS TO THE DAY OF THE SECOND BIOPSY AND THE DAY BEFORE AND AFTER IT.
*** PATIENTS IN WHICH CDCA INDUCED CONSTIPATION

Figure 22 Effect of CDCA treatment in gallstone patients on concentration of cAMP and cGMP in colonic mucosal biopsy specimens in relation to fecal frequency

– cAMP and cGMP – in association with the induced diarrhea (Figure 22).

Note also that there is a progressive decrease in the levels of both cyclic nucleotides, in association with diminution in the diarrhea. This phenomenon can be explained by a single pharmacological mechanism.

We treated 16 patients with 10 mg/kg-day UDCA, and we studied the concomitant changes in levels of cAMP in colonic biopsies. After 5, 7 and 10 days, there was a significant increase in the intracellular levels of cAMP but not cGMP (Figure 23).

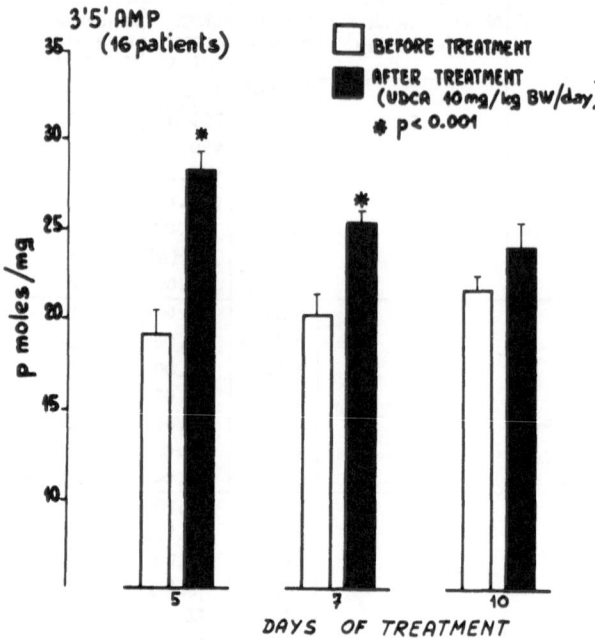

Figure 23 Effect of UDCA treatment at 10 mg/kg-day for 5 days (left), 7 days (centre), or 10 days (right) on the concentration of cAMP in colonic mucosal biopsy specimens

Thus, by contrast, cGMP is not affected by the administration of UDCA in the same dose and for the same duration of treatment (Figure 24).

To recapitulate, we propose the following: during CDCA treatment the diarrhea occurs because of a parallel increase of both nucleotides; our data suggest that the secretory mechanisms are not only dependent on cAMP. Treatment with UDCA induces significant increases in cAMP only and this occurs without diarrhea.

Caciagli: I should like to speak about some new experimental data that we have obtained in which our patients were pretreated with indomethacin. This treatment blocked the CDCA-induced side effect and prevented the increase of intracellular levels of both cyclic nucleotides. On the basis of this finding, the use of

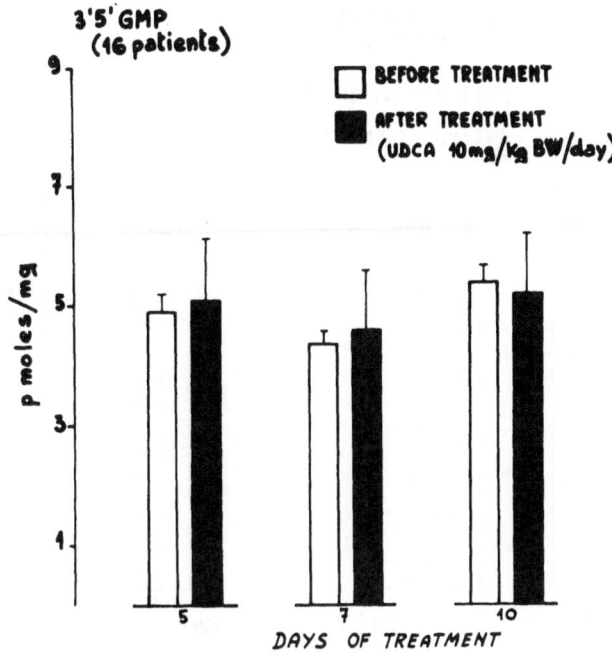

Figure 24 Effect of UDCA treatment at 10 mg/kg-day for 5 days (left), 7 days (centre), or 10 days (right) on the concentration of cGMP in colonic mucosal biopsy specimens

propranolol does not appear to be effective in blocking bile salt induced diarrhea (Coyne *et al.*, 1976). These findings appear to suggest that the secretory mechanisms of the human colonic mucosa are not only 3'5'AMP dependent. It seems likely in fact that the guanylate cyclase 3'5'GMP system is also involved in this mechanism (Figure 25).

Dowling: It is fair to say that this is only one of several postulated mechanisms whereby bile acids induce diarrhea. Furthermore, not everyone would agree with the statement about ß-blockers and the effectiveness of propanolol in treating bile acid mediated diarrhea.

Caciagli: Prostaglandins could be involved.

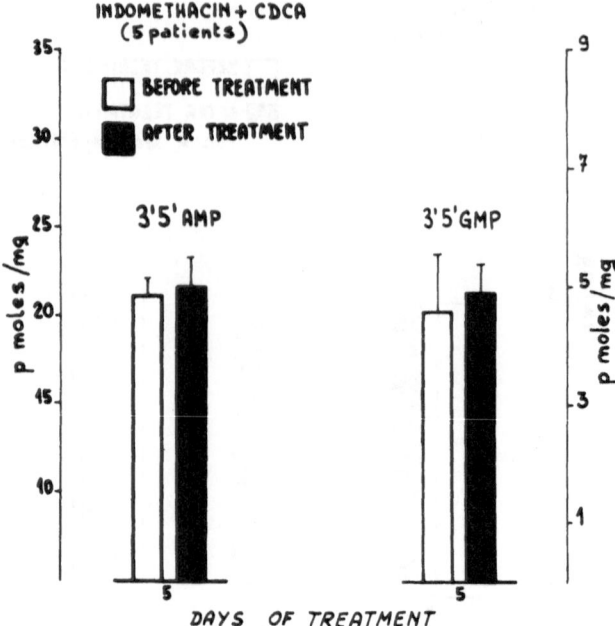

Figure 25   Effect of combined treatment with indomethacin + CDCA for 5 days on levels of cyclic nucleotides in colonic mucosal biopsy samples

Dowling: But to return to the role of cAMP, you found increased levels during UDCA therapy without diarrhea - is that correct?

Chadwick: Adenyl cyclase is situated on the basal membrane of the enterocyte, whereas guanyl cyclase is within the cell. Cell damage and non-specific activation of these enzymes could explain some of these findings, but the situation is a complex one.

Hofmann: We might speculate that when we feed UDCA, we mobilize the existing bile acid pool into the colon. The initial effects may not necessarily be caused by UDCA; they might reflect the consequence of more CDCA passing into the colon. Therefore, the mechanism of the initial effect is uncertain unless fecal bile acids are measured.

Roda, A: In our patients on UDCA, nobody had diarrhea.

Dowling: Perhaps, as a finale, we might think about where we should go in the field of gallstone dissolution and ursotherapy in the future, and whether we should use CDCA or UDCA - if, indeed, there is still a role for CDCA. But before doing so, does anyone want to comment on liver enzyme changes or hepatotoxicity of UDCA?

Stiehl: In the control study that we did in which we used the same patient as his own control, we observed elevated transaminase levels in four patients using a dose of 15 mg/kg. When we compared transaminases during ursotherapy with transaminases during chenotherapy we observed no increase with UDCA. So apparently, there seems to be a difference in toxicity.

Dowling: That certainly bears out the observations from Japan. Probably we have all been finding the same pattern of results: if so, we should not spend too long on it.

Does everybody find that hypertransaminasemia does not occur during UDCA therapy?

Roda, E: As you can see, nobody on UDCA therapy had an increase in the transaminase levels. However, only one patient in the CDCA group had an increased level of transaminase (Figure 26).

Roda, A: In the same controlled trial we measured serum bile acids by radioimmunoassay, specific for CDCA,

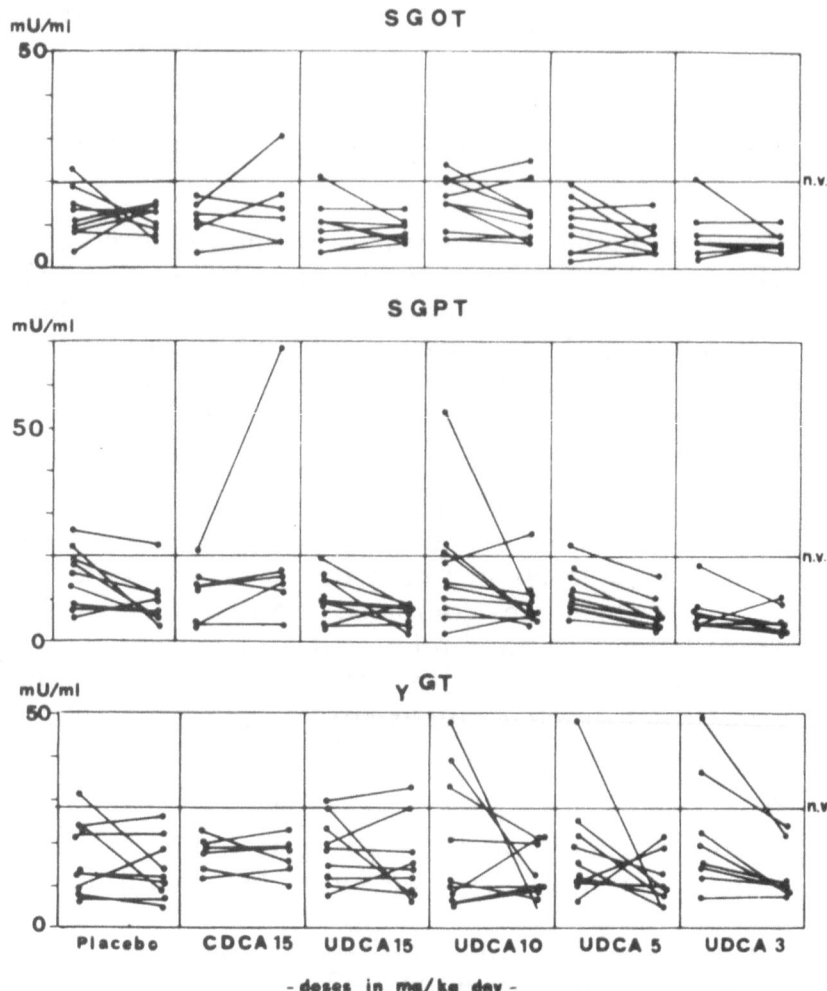

Figure 26 Serum levels of liver disease - associated enzymes before and after 3 months of treatment with UDCA, CDCA, or placebo

cholic acid, lithocholic acid, and UDCA conjugates developed by us (Figure 27). Studies on cross-reaction, parallelism and recovery to assess the reproducibility, precision, and accuracy have already been reported (Roda, A. *et al.*, 1977a; Roda, A. *et al.*, 1977b).

In the placebo group there were no changes during

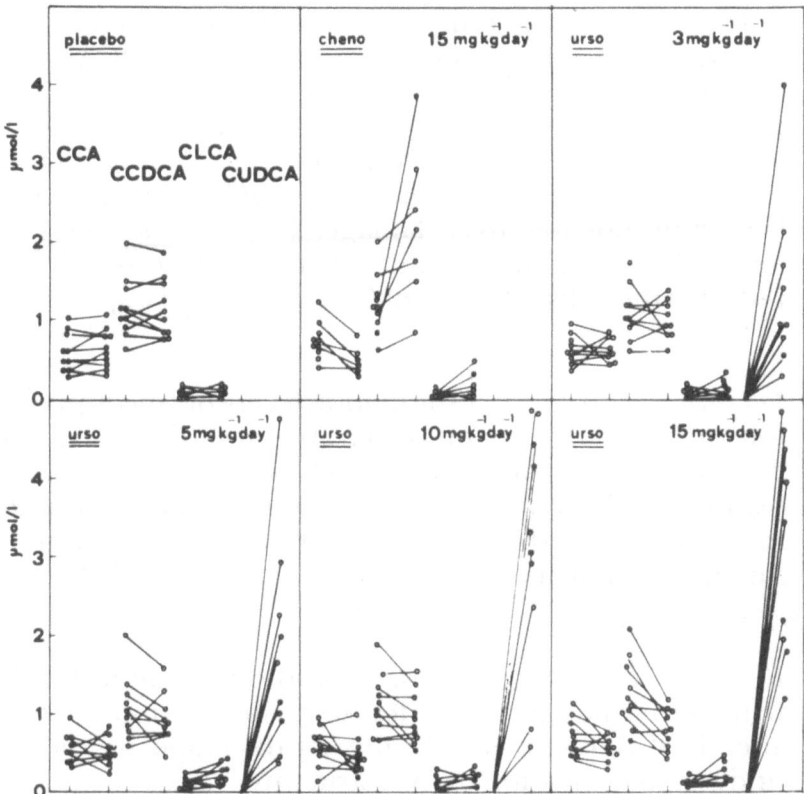

Figure 27 Fasting-state serum bile acid levels (μmol/l) in the placebo-chenodeoxycholic acid-ursodeoxycholic acid controlled trial before (left panel) and after (right two panels) 3 months of therapy. CCA = conjugated cholic acid; CCDCA = conjugated chenodeoxycholic acid; CLCA = conjugated lithocholic acid; CUDCA = conjugated ursodeoxycholic acid

treatment. CDCA was the predominant bile acid in serum, and lithocholic acid was present in a minimal amount. UDCA was not present. In the CDCA group, after therapy, CDCA increased significantly while the other bile acids fell. Lithocholic acid did not increase; total bile acids, before and after, did not increase significantly. In the UDCA group, UDCA was present after treatment and was dose related.

The increase in serum UDCA after ursotherapy was higher than the increase in serum CDCA after chenotherapy at the same doses. The other bile acids fell significantly, but were still present in minimal amounts. Total serum bile acids, before and after, did not increase significantly after UDCA and CDCA therapy, thus excluding possible liver damage. The increase in UDCA and CDCA in serum paralleled the increase in bile and reflected the redistribution of CDCA and UDCA pools.

Dowling: You are talking about levels of unconjugated bile acid in the serum when the intestine is full of exogenous free bile acids which are constantly being reabsorbed. You are not suggesting that in this situation the finding of high unconjugated bile acid in the serum is a manifestation of liver toxicity, are you?

Roda, E: No. In seven cases, we studied liver morphology with light and electron microscopy before and 1 month after UDCA treatment (12 mg/kg-day), and we did not find any modification in liver structure.

Dowling: Aren't the elevated serum bile acid levels (of CDCA and UDCA) merely a physiological phenomenon reflecting alterations in the composition of biliary bile acids rather than a manifestation of liver toxicity?

Roda, E: I did not mean to suggest that these changes in serum bile acid levels indicate hepatotoxicity.

Hofmann: And it is what we would expect. Serum bile acids are similar to the biliary bile acids, but there is distortion because they have different first-pass clearances (Schalm *et al.*, 1978).

Dowling: Dr Roda's group seems to have the most patients, and also he compared CDCA and UDCA. Did he find a difference in the level of serum enzymes between the two groups? Were there patients who showed toxicity on CDCA?

Roda, E: Not toxicity. We have observed only one case of elevation of transaminases in the CDCA group.

Fromm: Does Professor Dowling believe that it is well documented that CDCA causes elevated transaminase levels? Were the studies well enough controlled? We have not found more transaminase elevations before treatment than during administration of CDCA (Fromm *et al.*, 1975).

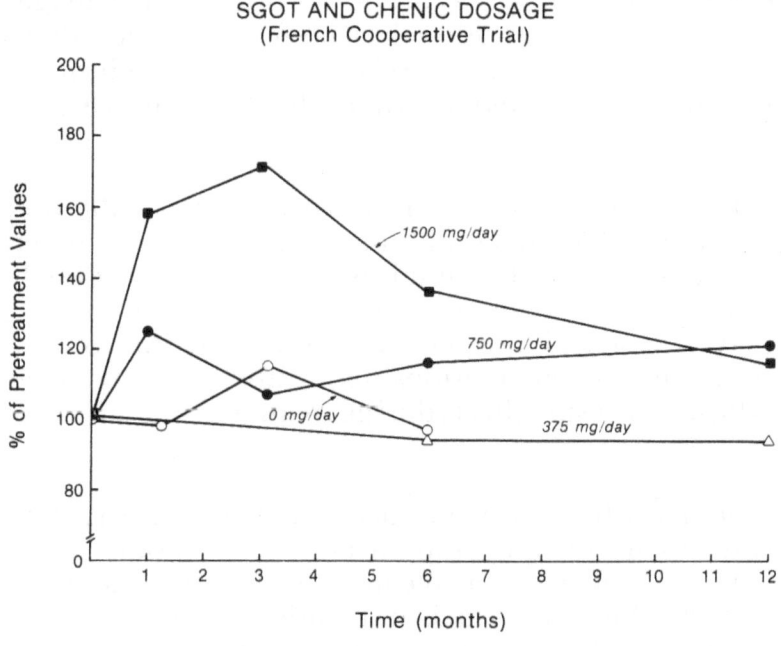

Figure 28 Time course of levels of SGOT in relation to CDCA dose in the French cooperative trial (data of Gerolami *et al.* (1977). *Digestion,* **16**, 299-308.

Dowling: There are a large number of published papers where the majority of investigators find a modest rise in serum transaminase levels in about 30% (approximately) of patients.

Hofmann: The data from the French cooperative trial (Gerolami *et al.*, 1977), which were published last year are unequivocal (Figure 28). There is a dose-related, transient transaminasemia in patients receiving CDCA. Whether this is hepatotoxicity, depends on one's definition. The elevated transaminase levels are not associated with morphological abnormalities. Therefore, it seems to me that these transaminase elevations are false 'positives', possibly related to increased membrane permeability. However, no other drug has as yet been noticed to do this.

In my own opinion, aspirin may well turn out also to cause transaminase elevations without liver damage. In general, the assumption has been in the past that the elevated transaminase levels were a true indication of hepatotoxicity. This seems not to be true with CDCA.

Dowling: That may well be true, but we really do not know what to make of this modest increase in serum transaminase levels. Certainly we must say that the bulk of evidence suggests that CDCA is not hepatotoxic.

We must call the meeting to an end. Are there any comments or observations about any unusual or novel symptoms or side effects during treatment?

Hofmann: It must be pointed out that CDCA is a major constituent of the enterohepatic circulation in man, whereas UDCA is not. We may see unusual side effects of UDCA. We must watch our patients closely. We must attempt to decide what is cause and effect and what is coincidence. At the first cheno workshop, someone reported that a patient's acne had strikingly improved during CDCA ingestion. I think that this was coincidental, but we must still look for unusual things, because never before in the history of enterohepatology has the composition of the circulatory bile acids been changed so markedly.

References

Adler, T. D., Bennion, L. J., Duane, W. C. *et al.* (1975). Effects of low dose chenodeoxycholic acid feeding on biliary lipid metabolism. *Gastroenterology*, **68**, 326-334.

Ashizawa, S., Ishi N., Ishihara, H. *et al.* (1977). Clinical study of gallstone dissolution with ursodeoxycholic acid. *Igaku no ayumi (Progress in Medicine)* **101**, 922-936. (Japanese).

van Berge Henegouwen, G. P., Hofmann, A. F. and Gaginella, T. S. (1977a). Pharmacology of chenodeoxycholic acid. I. Pharmaceutical properties. *Gastroenterology*, **73**, 291-299.

van Berge Henegouwen, G. P. and Hofmann, A. F. (1977b). Pharmacology of chenodeoxycholic acid. II. Absorption and metabolism in man. *Gastroenterology*, **73**, 300-309.

Binder, H. J., Filburn, C. and Volpe, B. T. (1975). Bile salt alteration of colonic electrolyte transport: Role of cyclic adenosine monophosphate. *Gastroenterology*, **68**, 503-508.

Calcraft, B., LaRusso, N. F., Hofmann, A. F. *et al.* (1975). Development of a simple, safe, bile acid clearance test: The radio-cholate clearance test. *Gastroenterology*, **69**, 812 (abstract).

Carey, M. C., Mazer, N. A. and Benedek, G. B. (1977). Novel physical-chemical properties of ursodeoxycholic acid (UDCA) and its conjugates: Relevance to gallstone dissolution in man. *Gastroenterology*, **72**, 1036 (abstract).

Chadwick, V. S., Phillips, S. F. and Hofmann, A. F. (1977). Measurements of intestinal permeability using low molecular weight polyethylene glycols (PEG 400). II. Application to studies of normal and abnormal permeability states in man and animals. *Gastroenterology*, **73**, 247-251.

Chadwick, V. S., Gaginella, T. S., Debongnie, J. C. *et al.* (1976b). Mucosal epitheliolysis: A mechanism for the increased colonic permeability induced by dihydroxy bile acids. *Gut*, **17**, 816 (abstract).

Chadwick, V. S., Gaginella, T. S., Debongnie, J.-C. *et al.* (1976c). Different effects of chenodeoxycholic and ursodeoxycholic acids on colonic secretion, permeability and morphology. *Gastroenterology*, **71**, 900 (abstract).

Conley, D. R., Coyne, M. J., Bonorris, G. G. *et al.* (1976). The mechanism of bile acid diarrhea: Stimulation of colonic adenylate cyclase and secretion in the rabbit. *Am. J. Dig. Dis.*, **21**, 453-458.

Coyne, M. J., Bonorris, G. G., Chung, A. *et al.* (1976). Inhibition by propranolol of bile acid stimulation of rabbit colonic adenylate cyclase in vitro. *Gastroenterology*, **71**, 68-71.

Danzinger, R. G., Hofmann, A. F., Schoenfield, L. J. *et al.* (1972). Dissolution of cholesterol gallstones by chenodeoxycholic acid. *N. Engl. J. Med.*, **286**, 1-8.

Debongnie, J.-C. and Phillips, F. C. (1977). Colonic function and diarrhea. *Gastroenterology*, **72**, 1046 (abstract).

Einarsson, K., Hellström, K. and Kallner, M. (1974). Influence of deoxycholic acid feeding on the elimination of cholesterol in normolipemia subjects. *Clin. Sci. Mol. Med.*, **47**, 425-433.

Eneroth, P., Gordon, B., Ryhage, R. *et al.* (1966). Identification of mono- and dihydroxy bile acids in human feces by gas-liquid chromatography and mass spectrometry. *J. Lipid Res.*, **7**, 511-523.

Erlinger, S., Poupon, R., Glasinovic, J. C. *et al.* (1977). Hepatic uptake, storage and biliary transport maximum of bile acids in the dog. In: G. Paumgartner and A. Stiehl (eds.), *Bile Acid Metabolism in Health and Disease.* pp. 107-112. (Lancaster: MTP Press Limited).

Fedorowski, T., Salen, G., Colallilo, A. *et al.* (1977). Metabolism of ursodeoxycholic acid in man. *Gastroenterology*, **73**, 1131-1137.

Ferrari, A., Scholastico, C. and Beretta, L. (1977). On the mechanism of cholic acid 7α-dehydroxylation by a *Chlostridium difermentans* cell-free extract. *FEBS Letters*, **75**, 166-167.

Fromm, H., Holz-Slomczyk, M., Zobl, H. *et al.* (1975). Studies of liver function and structure in patients with gallstones before and during treatment with chenodeoxycholic acid. *Acta Hepato-Gastroent.*, **22**, 359-369.

Fromm, H., Erbler, H. C., Eschler, A. *et al.* (1976). Alterations of bile acid metabolism during treatment with chenodeoxycholic acid. Studies of the role of the appearance of ursodeoxycholic acid in the dissolution of gallstones. *Klin. Wochenschr.*, **54**, 1125-1131.

Fromm, H., Farivar, S., Carlson, G. L. *et al.* (1977). Hepatic formation of ursodeoxycholic acid from 7-ketolithocholic acid in man. *Gastroenterology*, **73**, 1221 (abstract).

Fromm, H., Farivar, S., Carlson, G. L. *et al.* (1978). Metabolism and enterohepatic circulation of an important secondary bile acid in man. *Gastroenterology*, **74**, 1123 (abstract).

Gerolami, A., Sarles, H., Brette, R. *et al.* (1977). Controlled trial of chenodeoxycholic therapy for radiolucent gallstones: A multicenter study. *Digestion*, **16**, 299-307.

Grundy, S. M., Ahrens, E. H. Jr and Miettinen, T. A. (1965). Quantitative isolation and gas-liquid chromatographic analysis of total fecal bile acids. *J. Lipid Res.*, **6**, 397-410.

Hegardt, F. G. and Dam, H. (1971). The solubility of cholesterol in aqueous solution of bile salts and lecithin. *Z. Ernähr.*, **10**, 223-233.

Hellström, K. and Sjövall, J. (1960). Metabolism of chenodeoxycholic acid in the rabbit. Bile acids and steroids 104. *Acta Chem. Scand.*, **14**, 1763-1769.

Hislop, I. G., Hofmann, A. F. and Schoenfield, L. J. (1967). Determinants of the rate and site of bile acid absorption in man. *J. Clin. Invest.*, **46**, 1070-1071 (abstract).

Hofmann, A. F. and Paumgartner, G. (1975). *Chenodeoxycholic Acid Therapy of Gallstones: Update 1975.* (Stuttgart, New York: F. K. Schattauer Verlag).

Hofmann, A. F., Thistle, J. L., Klein, P. D. *et al.* (1978). Chenotherapy for gallstones. II. Induced changes in bile composition and gallstone response. *J. Am. Med. Assoc.*, **239**, 1145-1147.

Holzbach, R. T., Marsh, M., Olszewski, M. *et al.* (1973). Cholesterol solubility in bile: Evidence that supersaturated bile is frequent in healthy man. *J. Clin. Invest.*, **52**, 1467-1479.

Igimi, H., Noriyuki, T., Yuichi, I. *et al.* (1977). Ursodeoxycholic — in vitro cholesterol solubility and changes of composition of human gallbladder-bile after oral treatment. *Life Sci.*, **21**, 1373-1380.

Iser, J. H., Murphy, G. M. and Dowling, R. H. (1977). Speed of change in biliary lipids and bile acids with chenodeoxycholic acid - is intermittent therapy feasible? *Gut*, **18**, 7-15.

Johnston, C. G. and Nakayama, F. (1957). Solubility of cholesterol and gallstones in metabolic material. *Arch. Surg.*, **75**, 436-442.

Kwan, K. H., Higuchi, W. I., Molokhia, A. M. *et al.* (1977). Dissolution kinetics of cholesterol in simulated bile. I. Influence of bile acid type and concentration, bile acid/lecithin ratio, and added electrolyte. *J. Pharm. Sci.*, **66**, 1094-1101.

LaRusso, N. F., Hoffman, N. E. and Hofmann, A. F. (1974). Validity of using 2,4-^{3}H-labeled bile acids to study bile acid kinetics in man. *J. Lab. Clin. Med.*, **84**, 759-765.

LaRusso, N. F., Szczepanik, P. A., Hofmann, A. F. *et al.* (1977). The effect of deoxycholic acid ingestion on bile acid metabolism and biliary lipid secretion in normal subjects. *Gastroenterology*, **72**, 132-140.

Lindstedt, S. (1957). The turnover of cholic acid in man. *Acta Physiol. Scand.*, **40**, 1-9.

Low-Beer, T. S. and Pomare, E. W. (1975). Can colonic bacterial metabolites predispose to cholesterol gall stone? *Br. Med. J.*, **1**, 438-440.

Mahowald, T. A., Yin, M. W., Matschiner, J. T. *et al.* (1958). VIII. Metabolism of 7-ketolithocholic acid-24-C^{14} in the rat. *J. Biol. Chem.*, **230**, 581-588.

Makino, I., Shinozaki, K., Yoshino, K. *et al.* (1975). Dissolution of cholesterol gallstones by ursodeoxycholic acid. *Jap. J. Gastroent.*, **72**, 690-702.

Maton, P. N., Murphy, G. M. and Dowling, R. H. (1977). Ursodeoxycholic acid treatment of gallstones - dose response study and possible mechanism of action. *Lancet*, **2**, 1297-1301.

Metzger, A. L., Heymsfield, S. and Grundy, S. M. (1972). The lithogenic index - A numerical expression for the relative lithogenicity of bile. *Gastroenterology*, **62**, 499-501 (Letter to Editor).

Nakagawa, S., Makino, I., Ishizaki, T. *et al.* (1977). Dissolution of cholesterol gallstones by ursodeoxycholic acid. *Lancet*, **2**, 367-369.

Ng, P. Y., Allan, R. N. and Hofmann, A. F. (1977). Suitability of 11,12-^{3}H$_2$-chenodeoxycholic acid and 11,12-^{3}H$_2$-lithocholic acid for isotope dilution studies of bile acid metabolism in man. *J. Lipid Res.*, **18**, 753-758.

Ponz de Leon, M. and Dowling, R. H. Clinical pharmacology of oral chenodeoxycholic acid (CDCA). *Gut*, **18**, A976 (abstract).

Reichen, J., Preisig, R. and Paumgartner, G. (1977). Influence of chemical structure on hepatocellular uptake of bile acids. In: G. Paumgartner and A. Stiehl (eds.), *Bile Acid Metabolism in Health and Disease*. pp. 113-123. (Lancaster: MTP Press Limited).

Roda, A., Roda, E., Festi, D. *et al.* (1977a). A radioimmunoassay of primary bile acid conjugates in human serum. *La Ricerca Clin. Lab.*, **7**, 163-178.

Roda, A. Roda, E., Aldini, R. *et al.* (1977b). Development, validation and application of a single-tube radioimmunoassay for cholic and chenodeoxycholic conjugated bile acids in human serum. *Clin. Chem.*, **23**, 2107-2113.

Roda, A., Roda, E., Aldini, R. *et al.* (1977c). Determination of $^{14}CO_2$ in breath and ^{14}C in stool after oral administration of cholyl-1-^{14}C glycine: Clinical application. *Clin. Chem.*, **23**, 2127.

Roda, E., Aldini, R., Mazzella, G. *et al.* (1978). Enterohepatic circulation of bile acids after cholecystectomy. *Gut* (in press).

Salen, G., Tint, G. S., Eliav, B. *et al.* Increased formation of ursodeoxycholic acid in patients treated with chenodeoxycholic acid. *J. Clin. Invest.*, **53**, 612-621.

Samuelsson, B. (1959). On the metabolism of chenodeoxycholic acid in the rat. *Acta Chem. Scand.*, **13**, 976-983.

Samuelsson. B., (1960). On the mechanism of the biological formation of deoxycholic acid from cholic acid. *J. Biol. Chem.*, **235**, 361.

Schalm, S. W., LaRusso, N. F., Hofmann, A. F., *et al.* Enterohepatic circulatory dynamics of primary bile acid conjugates in health and disease. *Gut* (in press).

Shaeiwitz, J. A., Evans, D. F., Cussler, E. L. *et al.* (1977). Cholesterol stone dissolution kinetics. *Clin. Res.*, **25**, 317A (abstract).

Stiehl, A., Czygan, P., Kommerell, B. *et al.* Urso vs cheno: A comparison of their effects on bile acid and bile lipid composition in patients with cholesterol gallstones. *Gastroenterology (in press)*.

Stiehl, A., Raedsch, R., Regula, M. *et al.* (1975). Zur Behandlung von Patienten mit Cholesteringallensteinen mit Chenodesoxycholsäure: Veränderungen im Gallensaurenstoffwechsel. *Inn. Med.*, **2**, 13-18.

Tangedahl, T. N., Matseshe, J. W., Thistle, J. L. *et al.* (1977). Plant sterols increase effectiveness of chenodeoxycholic acid therapy in lowering cholesterol saturation of fasting-state bile in patients with radiolucent gallstones. *Gastroenterology*, **72**, 1138 (abstract).

Tangedahl, T. N., Hofmann, A. F. and Kottke, B. A. Effects of primary bile acid ingestion alone or in combination with plant sterols on serum cholesterol levels, biliary lipid secretion, and bile acid metabolism in patients with type IIa hyperlipoproteinemia. *J. Lipid Res.* (in press).

Thistle, J. L. and Schoenfield, L. J. (1971). Induced alterations in composition of bile of persons having cholelithiasis. *Gastroenterology*, **61**, 488-496.

Thistle, J. L., Turcotte, J., Ott, B. J. *et al.* (1978). Ursodeoxycholic acid unsaturates bile at a lower dose than chenodeoxycholic acid. *Gastroenterology*, **74**, 1103 (abstract).

Thomas, P. J. and Hofmann, A. F. (1973). A simple calculation of the lithogenic index: Expressing biliary lipid composition on rectangular coordinates. *Gastroenterology*, **65**, 698-700 (Letter to Editor).